Changing

The Teamcare Valleys Experience

Changing Primary Health Care
The Teamcare Valleys Experience

Edited by

Rosamund Bryar *MPhil B Nurs RGN RHV NDN RM, Cert Ed (FE)*
Professor of Community Healthcare Nursing Practice
School of Health
University of Hull/Hull and Holderness Community Health NHS Trust

and

Bill Bytheway *BSc, PhD*
Lecturer in Sociology
University of Wales, Swansea

Blackwell
Science

© 1996 by
Blackwell Science Ltd
Editorial Offices:
Osney Mead, Oxford OX2 0EL
25 John Street, London WC1N 2BL
23 Ainslie Place, Edinburgh EH3 6AJ
238 Main Street, Cambridge
  Massachusetts 02142, USA
54 University Street, Carlton
  Victoria 3053, Australia

Other Editorial Offices:
Arnette Blackwell SA
  224, Boulevard Saint Germain
  75007 Paris, France

Blackwell Wissenschafts-Verlag GmbH
  Kurfürstendamm 57
  10707 Berlin, Germany

  Zehetnergasse 6
  A-1140 Wien
  Austria

First published 1996

Set in 10 on 12 pt Palatino
by DP Photosetting, Aylesbury, Bucks
Printed and bound in Great Britain by
Hartnolls Ltd., Bodmin, Cornwall

The Blackwell Science logo is a
trade mark of Blackwell Science Ltd,
registered at the United Kingdom
Trade Marks Registry

DISTRIBUTORS

Marston Book Services Ltd
PO Box 269
Abingdon
Oxon OX14 4YN
(*Orders:* Tel: 01235·465500
     Fax: 01235 465555)

USA
Blackwell Science, Inc.
238 Main Street
Cambridge, MA 02142
(*Orders:* Tel: 800 215-1000
     617 876-7000
     Fax: 617 492-5263)

Canada
Copp Clark, Ltd
2775 Matheson Blvd East
Mississauga, Ontario
Canada, L4W 4P7
(*Orders:* Tel: 800 263-4374
     905 238-6074)

Australia
Blackwell Science Pty Ltd
54 University Street
Carlton, Victoria 3053
(*Orders:* Tel: 03 9347 0300
     Fax: 03 9349 3016)

A catalogue record for this title
is available from the British Library

ISBN 0–632–03938–8

Library of Congress
Cataloging-in-Publication Data

Changing primary health care: the Teamcare
  Valleys experience/edited by Rosamund
  Bryar and Bill Bytheway.
     p.   cm.
  Includes bibliographical references and
index.
  ISBN 0–632–03938–8 (alk. paper)
  1. Primary health care—Wales—
Administration. 2. Health care teams—
Wales. I. Bryar, Rosamund. II. Bytheway,
Bill.
  [DNLM: 1. Primary Health Care—
organization & administration—Wales.
W 84.6 C4565 1996]
RA427.9.C48 1996
362.1′09429—dc20
DNLM/DLC
for Library of Congress   96-8525
                            CIP

Dedication

To Julian Tudor Hart, an inspiration to all those working to raise the health of the population of South Wales, and to all the primary health care teams working in the Valleys.

Early in the course of preparing this book, Chris Hoddell died. Chris was an enthusiastic collaborator with Teamcare Valleys and we greatly valued working with him. This book is also dedicated to his memory.

Contents

List of Contributors

Mary Ellen Brown   *BA (Hons), RGN, Diploma in Community Health Studies*, Health Visitor, Riverside Health Centre, Cardiff Community Healthcare NHS Trust, Merthyr Tydfil

Rosamund Bryar   *MPhil, B Nurs, RGN, RHV, NDN, RM, Cert Ed (FE)*, Professor of Community Healthcare Nursing Practice, School of Health, University of Hull/Hull and Holderness Community Health NHS Trust

Bill Bytheway   *BSc, PhD*, Lecturer in Sociology, University of Wales, Swansea

Lisa Coles   *RGN, RHV, BA*, Health Visitor (Research), Rhondda NHS Trust, Mid Glamorgan

Gwen Davies   *SRN, ONC, RHV, DipPH, Cert Ed*, Lecturer, Neath College, West Glamorgan

Patricia Davies   *MPhil, DipN (Lond), RNT, RMN*, Research Nurse, Powys Health Care NHS Trust, Training and Education Department, Mid Wales Hospital

Lyn Fisk   *SRN, HV, FET Cert*, Health Visitor, Bridgend and District NHS Trust

Peter Ganesh   *HND, DMS*, Practice Manager, Dowlais Medical Practice, Merthyr Tydfil

Jennie Gill   *RGN, RHV, Cert Ed (FE)*, Practice Based Team Facilitator, Cardiff Community Healthcare NHS Trust, Merthyr Tydfil

Beth Griffiths   *RGN, RM, Cert in Prof Practice*, Practice Health Facilitator, Amman Valley Medical Practice, Gwaun-cae-Gurwen, West Glamorgan

Chris Hoddell   *MBBCh, MRCGP, DRCOG*, formerly General Practitioner, Market Street Practice, Tonyfelin Surgery, Caerphilly, Mid Glamorgan

Helen Houston *DRCOG, MRCGP, DCH, MD,* Senior Lecturer, Department of General Practice, University of Wales College of Medicine, Cardiff

Robert Jones *MRCGP,* General Practitioner, Market Street Practice, Tonyfelin Surgery, Caerphilly, Mid Glamorgan

Paul Lewis *RMN, RCNT, FETC, CPN Cert,* Behaviour Nurse Therapist, Mental Health Resource Centre, Ystradgynlais, Powys

Rose Mary Marx *SRN, RM, DAM,* Community Midwife, Llanelli Dinefwr NHS Trust, Carmarthenshire

Rachel Pritchard *MPH, MRSH, RN, ONC, NDNC, CMS, RNT (District Nursing), PGCE (FE),* Clinical Services Manager (Adult and Elderly Community, and Community Hospital), Glanhafren NHS Trust, Gwent

Harold Proctor *RMN, CPN Cert,* Community Psychiatric Nurse, Ystradgynlais, Powys

Christine Rees *RN, RM, NDN, Dip DN,* District Nursing Sister, Blaina, Gwent Community Health NHS Trust

Julie Slater *RGN, BA (Hons),* Diploma in Health Education, Research Scientist, Institute of Work Psychology, University of Sheffield

Ajay Thapar *BSc (Hons), MBChB, DCH, DRCOG, MRCGP,* Lecturer in General Practice, Department of General Practice, University of Manchester

Andrea Thomas *BSc, RGN RM, RHV, HVT,* Health Visitor, North Glamorgan NHS Trust

Carl Venn *BSc, MBChB, DRCOG, MRCGP,* Principal in General Practice, Abertillery, Gwent

Brian Wallace *MB BS, FRCGP,* formerly Director, Teamcare Valleys, and formerly Senior Lecturer in General Practice, University of Wales College of Medicine

Diane Wallis *MBChB, MRCGP,* Senior Registrar in Public Health Medicine, South Staffordshire Health Authority, Stafford

Duncan Williams *MBBCh, MRCGP, DRCOG,* General Practitioner, Gwaun-cae-Gurwen, West Glamorgan

Stephanie Williams *BA, MA (Leeds), MIHSM,* Director, Valleys Health Group, Hensol Hospital, Pontyclun, Mid Glamorgan

Foreword

I am pleased to have been associated with Teamcare Valleys, albeit at a distance, and to be invited to write this Foreword for *Changing Primary Health Care: The Teamcare Valleys Experience*.

The Teamcare Valleys project was launched in 1990 as part of the Welsh Office Programme for the Valleys. The aims of the project were to: (a) make a significant contribution to the sponsorship of better health in the valleys as well as helping to deliver treatment services; (b) provide support of direct operational value to assist the delivery of primary care in the valleys; (c) provide a source of professional, research, managerial and entrepreneurial expertise to place at the disposal of primary care practitioners in the valleys; (d) promote the positive benefits of multi- and interdisciplinary team working in primary care (for the community and practitioners alike) through training and other practical measures; (e) sustain and complement the commitment of all those involved in primary care throughout the area.

The activities of Teamcare Valleys were many and varied, but focused on the importance of support for the multidisciplinary teams providing primary health care in the South Wales Valleys. The project was an innovative means of providing such support.

This interesting book is a chronicle of the work of many individuals. The content reflects the variety of topics explored through the project and their impact on the development of individuals, primary health care teams and services in the valleys. The results have been presented to illustrate the management aspects of developments, the potential for improvement through audit, the role of education, the importance of identifying community needs and the value of teamwork, which powered this project.

The experience of Teamcare Valleys' participants and supporters has been captured by the editors in a way that encourages and promotes further interest and development. The ideas are relevant to primary care development in both cities and rural areas. *Changing Primary Health Care: The Teamcare Valleys Experience* is a useful contribution to the literature and is recommended reading for all those with an interest in promoting primary health care.

Marion P. Bull *OBE* Chief Nursing Officer, Welsh Office

Preface

This book arises out of a major team effort – the team concept has operated at all sorts of levels: between institutions, between departments within institutions, between different professional groups, between primary health care teams in different parts of South Wales, between people committed to the development of primary health care in different parts of Britain and other parts of the world, and between a wide range of individuals who actively and energetically worked for this initiative called Teamcare Valleys (TCV). Teamcare Valleys was a multi-faceted Primary Health Care (PHC) development project initiated and funded by the Welsh Office for three years with the remit to help develop primary health care in the South Wales Valleys. There are unique features of TCV and of the South Wales Valleys, but there are also many similarities between issues facing PHC practitioners in South Wales and elsewhere. In parts of the country which may be somewhat flatter than South Wales, geographical barriers, town, city and village boundaries and community loyalties have similar influences on the development of PHC.

The dominant feeling we have in reflecting back on the experience is that of excitement: the excitement that the project generated and the willingness of all sorts of people to become embroiled in collaborative, inter-agency, inter-professional and inter-team, teamwork. We have little doubt ourselves that TCV succeeded in contributing to the process of change in PHC in South Wales, for the benefit of all. Lessons from TCV have already been applied in PHC projects in other parts of the country and it is hoped that publication of this book will lead to the further application and testing of methods used in TCV in other PHC projects.

Change continues, and during the preparation of this book for publication health authorities and FHSAs have merged, and local authorities have changed their names and their boundaries. Within the book we have retained the terms current between 1990 and 1993 when referring to activities during that time, but we have used current authority titles in sections that make recommendations for future action.

Rosamund Bryar and Bill Bytheway

Acknowledgements

There are many people and organisations to whom we owe thanks. We appreciate that TCV happened only because certain people in the Welsh Office and the University of Wales College of Medicine had the imagination to make it happen. We are greatly indebted to them. Likewise this book could not have been produced but for the efforts of hundreds of people working in primary health care teams in South Wales. All our past colleagues at TCV (listed in Appendix 1) have contributed directly or indirectly to this book. We hope they will consider it a worthy outcome of the team as a whole.

We are greatly indebted to Peter Elwood, who supported the whole operation, and to Brian Wallace, TCV Director, through whose patient support and encouragement the projects reported in this book came to fruition. We are grateful to Guy Lewis for the map, to Peter Gill for the photographs and to the PHCT members and patients who feature in some of them. In the production of this book we have valued the advice of Lisa Field, Teresa Heapy, Sarah-Kate Powell and Griselda Campbell of Blackwell Science, and in Swansea we extend thanks to Sheila Morgan for her secretarial help and to Chris Weeks of Babbage Design who provided technical support and unflagging bonhomie.

List of Abbreviations

CHC	Community Health Council
CME	Continuing Medical Education
COSHH	Control of Substances Hazardous to Health Regulations
CPN	Community Psychiatric Nurse
DGH	District General Hospital
DHA	District Health Authority
DoH	Department of Health
DySSSy	Dynamic Standard Setting System
FHSA	Family Health Services Authority
FPC	Family Practitioner Committee
GP	General Practitioner
HA	Health Authority
HbAlc	Glycated haemoglobin, a standard measure of blood glucose levels
HMSO	Her Majesty's Stationery Office
IPS	Interpersonal Skills
LEs	Life events
LMC	Local Medical Committee
MAAG	Medical Audit Advisory Group
MCQ	Multiple Choice Questionnaire
NHS	National Health Service
NHSE	National Health Service Executive
NHSME	National Health Service Management Executive
NVQ	National Vocational Qualification
OSI	Occupational Stress Indicator
PGEA	Postgraduate Education Allowance
PHC	Primary Health Care
PHCT	Primary Health Care Team

PREPP	Post-Registration Education and Practice Project
PRP	Practice Receptionist Training Programme
RCGP	Royal College of General Practitioners
RCN	Royal College of Nursing
RIDDOR	Reporting of Injuries, Disease and Dangerous Occurrences Regulations
RPS	Repeat Prescription System
SPSS	Statistical Package for the Social Sciences
TCV	Teamcare Valleys
UKCC	United Kingdom Central Council for Nursing, Midwifery and Health Visiting
UWCM	University of Wales College of Medicine
WHO	World Health Organization
WHPF	Welsh Health Planning Forum
WNB	Welsh National Board for Nursing, Midwifery and Health Visiting

Introduction

I was delighted when I was asked by the Welsh Office to chair the Steering Committee for the initiative that became Teamcare Valleys (TCV). Having spent 30 years in research within a Medical Research Council unit, I was glad to be given a chance to have an input into primary health care. The potential for the enrichment of the lives of primary health care workers by TCV was immediately obvious, and I reminisced that if only there had been the chance of involvement in research or some more academic activity during my own days in general practice, I might have stayed in general practice and my career might have been very different.

The idea behind the TCV initiative developed and changed greatly, and whoever first suggested the idea might not have recognised what eventually emerged. There was, however, more than a spark of genius in the germ of the idea of a multi-disciplinary team that would work alongside primary health care workers in a deprived and depressed area, generating interest and stimulating morale, and evaluating medical, nursing and other actions. Acknowledgement should go to Brian Wallace, Director of the initiative, who took what was little more than a concept and turned it into a dynamic, applied and widespread enterprise.

The concept of teamwork was central to TCV, not simply in its message, but also in its own structure and management. Hence both the management team and the fellows were drawn from a number of disciplines, and their base adjacent to the Valleys – the target area – became a hive of argument, discussion and planning. In all there were 36 fellows, and their projects led to the involvement of workers in over

90% of the health care teams within the target area. All this is clear from both the authorship and the content of the various chapters, and this bears testimony to the lateral thinking that characterised every level of the initiative.

The Steering Committee set up for the TCV project drew members from a wide range of NHS staff, with a strong Welsh Office presence in the background. In this way, the working of the group was controlled to maintain the accountability of the Committee.

The book records a considerable volume of work and the fact that a relatively small team was able to initiate and complete these studies is remarkable. The text demonstrates something of the potential of a multi-disciplinary team working alongside primary health care. What the volume does not attempt to evaluate is the enhancement of morale and the enrichment of the lives of the primary health care workers who became involved in the studies.

A mere three years was given to the Director to set up the scheme, appoint his management team and the fellows, and organise and complete the projects. MRC gives its research units five years between assessments once they are up and running. This volume records the remarkable achievements of those three years. The influence of TCV lives on – some of the fellows have remained in posts within the area, some have taken on wider responsibilities in the Valleys using skills acquired while with TCV, and others have moved into new areas of primary health care. Undoubtedly, those directly involved, as well as the readers of this book, will benefit from the knowledge and enthusiasm generated by the TCV initiative.

Professor Peter Elwood   *MD, FRCP, FFPHM*
Formerly Director of the MRC Epidemiology Unit, Cardiff

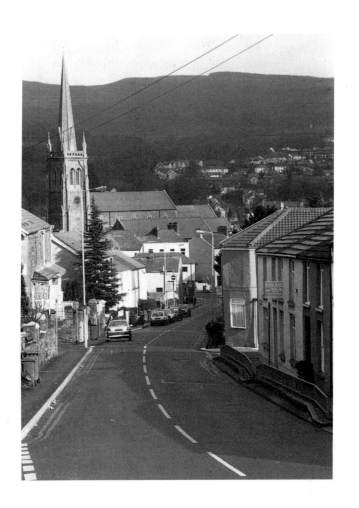

Chapter 1

Primary Health Care Development

Rosamund Bryar and Bill Bytheway

Introduction

In the 1995 William Pickles Lecture to the Royal College of General Practitioners, David Pendleton proposed the establishment of locally based professional development consultancy services for primary health care. The goal would be to: 'provide consultancy services to health care providers which maximise the impact of primary care on the health of the community' (Pendleton, 1995:380). This service, he argued, would be staffed by a range of professionals including representatives from the primary health care professions, education, research and other fields. It would work with practices on issues relating to service planning and audit, and would develop and provide continuing education. It would serve as a resource investigator, networker, facilitator, disseminator and communicator.

In Pendleton's view, such a service would bring together the academic and practice worlds, providing help and advice that was 'outside and separate' from the practice but at the same time was 'intimately involved with it'. In this way, he argued, the help that the service offered would be relevant and yet there would be 'no hidden agendas of its own' (p. 380). In short, in this important lecture, Pendleton makes a strong case for the provision of services that meet the developmental needs of local practices and primary health care teams.

If you are already familiar with the work of Teamcare Valleys (TCV) you may be forgiven for thinking that Pendleton was describing TCV (Wallace, 1993). In his description of a 'professional development consultancy service', he is outlining the essential elements and purposes of TCV which provided a focus for primary health care (PHC) development in the South Wales Valleys between 1990 and 1993. That the author of the William Pickles lecture could only describe a hypothetical PHC development unit, presumably unaware of TCV, demonstrates the long established problem of sharing and disseminating information in and about PHC and PHC development (Pearson & Spencer, in press).

TCV was involved in the dissemination of information about its activities but, as is illustrated in the following chapters, this was primarily to local practices and teams. As with so many developmental projects that have a local focus, wider dissemination was given a lower and longer-term priority. It is only now, some time after funding for the project has ended, and with no funds specifically allocated to dissemination, that this comprehensive account of the work of TCV has been brought together and published.

It is the purpose of this book to provide a description of the work of a unit of the kind outlined by Pendleton, one that endeavoured to meet the developmental needs of PHC practitioners and organisations. In preparing this book, we have had at the forefront of our minds those who have the task of establishing similar units. We hope they can learn from our experience. Each PHC development initiative has unique features and exists in a unique context. TCV was no exception in this respect, but we believe that lessons can be drawn from our experience which have a wider application, even to PHC settings in urban and rural areas which may share only a very few of the features of TCV or the South Wales Valleys.

The Report of the Inner City Task Force of the Royal College of General Practitioners (Lorentzon *et al.*, 1994:27) identifies four main obstacles to PHC practice in inner city areas: low patient education/ motivation/expectations; primary poverty/working class status; lack of time/overwork; and lack of funding/resources/PHC staff. At the beginning of TCV, information was collected from practitioners throughout the Valleys area on the problems they faced in providing PHC. The issues identified are very similar to those identified in the RCGP study: high workload; inappropriate use of services; reaching the difficult-to-reach members of the population; clinical problems; lack of teamwork; needs for staff training; and staff stress (Bytheway, 1991). The similarity of the issues supports our view that the description of the processes and outcomes of TCV may have wide relevance to the development of PHC in other areas.

TCV was part of a major government-funded programme aimed at the regeneration of the South Wales Valleys – an area of substantial deprivation. It was a three-year multidisciplinary initiative launched by the Welsh Office in conjunction with the University of Wales College of Medicine in 1990 – coincidentally, the year that the NHS introduced the first new Contract for general practice since 1966. The activities of TCV were focused on the PHC practices and PHC practitioners working in the Valleys. During the three years we explored new ways of creating opportunities for members of primary health care teams (PHCTs) to work with researchers, practice teachers and other practitioners, on projects and other activities which had as their ultimate aim the development of PHC in the area.

TCV therefore had a number of significant features. It was:

- government funded
- part of a wider political initiative
- working in an area of deprivation
- based in a university
- launched in 1990
- multidisciplinary
- multifaceted
- given the potential to try out new ideas, not just those guaranteed to work
- limited to three years.

In the following sections of this introductory chapter our aim is to describe the work of TCV and to place it in context. We also draw out some issues discussed in more detail elsewhere in the book that are of particular relevance to other PHC projects. First we begin with a review of PHC itself.

Why is primary health care development important?

Since 1978, stimulated by the priorities set by the World Health Organization, the main aim of health care service development throughout the world has been to re-orientate health services towards PHC. Economic pressures in less developed countries led to the early implementation of strategies designed to reduce health care costs, and to provide more locally based services which dealt with the common conditions prevalent in those areas.

In Britain the pattern of implementation has been different. PHC, general practice and community-based health care services have a long history and are associated with bureaucratic systems which are inimical to rapid change. Vested interests, political priorities and professional rivalries have all provided additional barriers to change (Owens *et al.*, 1995). However, even within this constrained and constraining system, change and a re-orientation of the health service towards PHC and services based in general practice has been evident. This change has been gathering momentum in Britain since the mid-1980s and particularly since the publication of *Working for Patients* (Secretary of State for Health, 1989), the policy document that established the contract culture in the new NHS. The speed of change in the years between 1990 and 1995 is illustrated by the emphasis now being placed on moves towards a primary care-led NHS (Bosanquet, 1995; NHSE, 1994). As with the changes in less developed countries, the main stimulus has been rising costs, and in particular the need to reduce the costs involved in providing services in secondary health care settings. The growing view in health service policy is that many services can be provided more conveniently and more effectively in PHC settings.

Success in switching services from the secondary sector to PHC depends on a number of factors, including the willingness of those in the secondary sector to actively engage in change, and the extent to which PHC service providers are able to meet the new demands being placed on them. Many of these demands require PHC practitioners to review their traditional roles and the role boundaries between the multiplicity of professional groups who are found working in PHC settings (Owens *et al.*, 1995). Interest in the process by which PHC practitioners can be helped to develop the necessary skills and knowledge has therefore been increasing in recent years. This can be illustrated by the huge rise in the numbers of facilitators employed in PHC. The concept of the facilitator was first developed in 1982, and by 1994 there were 304 in post working on specific projects and on general PHC development activities (Wilson, 1994).

There are, however, dangers in assuming that PHC means the same to everyone, and that everyone working in PHC is working at the same level, with the same resources and with the same opportunities for development. PHC is defined in different ways by different bodies. The World Health Organization definition focuses on the role of the community in PHC and the effects of involvement of the community in PHC on the: 'overall social and economic development of the country' (WHO, 1988:8). In Britain the focus is placed on PHC as the first level of contact that people have with the health care system, and emphasis is placed on the health care practitioners who are seen as the providers of PHC (Review of Community Nursing in Wales, 1987).

There are thus two major views of PHC. On the one hand PHC is viewed as being community-based and members of the population are seen as the first level of PHC, initiating and undertaking activities in relation to prevention, treatment and rehabilitation. On the other hand, PHC is viewed from the position of the health professions and is viewed as the first level of provision of services by health care practitioners. These opposing positions are further complicated by the public health perspective and community-orientated PHC which are characterised by the collection and utilisation of population level data about health status and health needs (Tollman, 1991). Either or both of these approaches may be utilised within a PHC system which takes the community as the starting point or which takes the PHC professionals as the starting point. Equally the utilisation of such data may be absent or very patchy in either system, as is evident in PHC services in the UK today (Standing Nursing and Midwifery Advisory Committee, 1995).

The development of a greater range of preventive, treatment and rehabilitation services in the community, including the transfer of services from acute settings, is gaining momentum (Vetter, 1995). We would argue that there is an urgent need for those in PHC and other parts of the health care system to debate their understanding of PHC and their views about the direction of development of PHC services (Tarimo & Webster, 1994). A shared view would then underpin PHC development activities undertaken in a particular area or by a particular team. PHC practice is inevitably changing and adequate support services are needed to enable all members of the PHCT to develop services that are as effective and efficient as possible. One mechanism for providing such support is via a PHC Research and Development Unit (Bryar, 1994a) such as TCV as described in this book.

Who are the PHC practitioners?

Alongside the debate as to the starting point of PHC there is another debate about the membership of the PHCT (Pringle, 1993). One view would be that all health care practitioners and all members of the community are potentially members of the PHCT. This approach, for example, influenced the teambuilding project discussed in Chapter 21 in which PHCTs attending workshops were required to bring with them a member of the community registered with the practice. Others view the PHCT in different ways. For example, some may view the PHCT as the GPs and those members of staff employed by the GPs including practice managers, receptionists, practice nurses and, increasingly, a wide range of therapists, counsellors and complementary therapists. Others consider that the PHCT also includes attached district nurses, health visitors, community psychiatric nurses, midwives, specialist nurses, social workers, pharmacists, other community workers and, in some cases, members of staff who are hospital based.

We held many discussions with practitioners throughout the Valleys on the definition of the PHCT. Consistently they described a picture of a multiplicity of teams working together rather than a picture of a single monolithic team. For example, a small team of a receptionist, district nurse, practice nurse and GP might work together on screening the over-75s, while a different team including another receptionist, health visitor, practice nurse and GP might work together on child health issues. A picture was thus drawn of a 'team' consisting of multiple small teams of people coming together in different combinations to meet the needs of different sections of the population. Equally consistently individuals commented on the difficulties of teamwork, some of which are common to other groups seeking to develop teams (West, 1994) but some of which may be more pronounced in PHC. Problems included the lack of understanding of roles and role boundaries which may inhibit the full utilisation of skills (Bryar, 1994b); physical separation of practitioners' bases; lack of time; lack of skills in organising team meetings; and problems caused by the employment of different team members by different organisations (an issue discussed in Chapter 17).

This discussion about the definition of the PHCT indicates the large number of different professional groups engaged in PHC practice. A third debate in PHC, which has developed in the 1990s, centres on the utilisation of the skills of PHCT members and challenges the established role boundaries found in PHC. Current and future health care needs require a flexible response from practitioners who are not restricted by traditional definitions of professional responsibilities (WHO, 1994; Owens *et al.*, 1995). Multidisciplinary working and education contributes to the understanding of roles and thus to a greater awareness of role overlap and the possibilities of change. Future definitions of the PHCT may thus be very different from current definitions.

For pragmatic reasons, the Steering Group for TCV decided to limit the definition of the PHCT to the core practice staff of general practitioners, practice manager, receptionists and practice nurse, and the attached staff of district nurses, health visitors, community psychiatric nurses and community midwives. Part way during the project pharmacists were added by the Steering Group to the definition of the PHCT.

TCV was thus concerned with members of what might be described as the traditional PHCT. The perception of the PHCT is constantly shifting and changing and for many of the people involved in TCV this restricted definition was a limiting factor in the work of TCV. However, as demonstrated in the following chapters, the breadth of work of TCV was very great just with the traditional PHCT members. We suggest that other projects whose work is not limited to the traditional PHCT members would need to ensure that they had staff members with the necessary experience to work with these other groups.

The South Wales Valleys

During the 1980s the government recognised the need to help the South Wales Valleys adjust to the decline of the coalmining industry. In 1988 Peter Walker, the then Secretary of State for Wales, launched the Valleys Initiative (Welsh Office, 1988). Its aim was to: 'build a new economy, repair the damaged environment and strengthen the social fabric of Valleys life' (Welsh Office, 1988:4). A wide-ranging programme of projects was initiated in the area including projects aimed at creating employment, upgrading the environment and transport, developing tourism activities (including, for example, the 1992 Ebbw Vale Garden Festival), refurbishing arts centres, and providing education and training. Also included were projects focused on the health of the Valleys population. Apart from TCV, these included hospital developments, day treatment centres, dental clinics, 'care of the elderly' projects and health promotion activities.

The Valleys of South Wales have a certain legendary quality and, as with all legends, it seems that everybody knows of the stereotype but little of the reality. There is an assumption, it often seems, that all the Valleys are fairly similar: steep-sided with long snake-like terraces of two-up, two-down houses broken periodically by a chapel or a school. The view itself captures the essence of a long tradition of community life based upon the mining industry, and drawing upon a range of powerful beliefs grounded in religion and relating to family, education and health (Jenkins & Edwards, 1990).

The boundaries of the area earmarked by the Welsh Office for the Valleys Initiative roughly followed those of the South Wales coalfield (see Appendices 2 and 3). The equivalence of 'Valleys' and 'coal' might be construed to imply that the area has a certain geographical consistency. In fact there are substantial differences, to the extent that it is dangerous to generalise about the Valleys as a whole. The physical geography of the area is important in that it determines to a large extent the pattern of travel, the isolation and the sense of place that dominates life in the Valleys. It affects the organisation of PHC services just as much as, for example, the pattern of shopping.

Overall there are 26 valleys. Starting in the east, there are the four Gwent valleys which include some of the narrowest and most inaccessible parts of the area. They are drained by rivers that flow southwards to meet the Bristol Channel at Newport. Next there are the five large valleys of Mid Glamorgan: Rhymney, Taff, Cynon, Rhondda Fach and Rhondda Fawr, interspersed by some smaller valleys. All the rivers of these valleys flow south-east towards Cardiff. West of these, the main valleys, the Neath and the Tawe, are broad-bottomed, less heavily populated and lead south-westwards to Swansea Bay. Between the Neath and the Rhondda Fawr, however, there are a series of smaller narrow 'cul-de-sac' valleys: the Ogmore, Garw, Llynfi and Afan, that flow towards Bridgend and Port Talbot. West of the Tawe, there are the Amman and Gwendraeth Valleys meandering through the rolling Dyfed hills to meet the sea in Carmarthen Bay.

About 700 000 people live in this area – a quarter of the population of Wales and equivalent to a city the size of Manchester. They are distributed fairly evenly throughout the Valleys, but with the greater densities in the east. There is no natural centre and few of the main towns: Pontypool, Ebbw Vale, Tredegar, Merthyr Tydfil, Aberdare, Pontypridd, Caerphilly and Maesteg, serve as centres for more than two or three Valleys. More significantly the cities of Swansea and

Cardiff are close but outside the area, as are the large towns of Abergavenny, Newport, Bridgend and Neath. Most of the district general hospitals that serve the area are in these neighbouring towns and cities. So, despite the shared identity created by the word 'Valleys', the population is fragmented geographically and served primarily by regional centres in the adjacent coastal area.

The coastal dominance is reflected in the transport systems. The main railway line and the M4 motorway, connecting South Wales to the rest of Britain, pass through or close to Swansea, Bridgend, Cardiff and Newport. Paralleling this is the Heads of the Valleys, a trunk road that connects the Neath Valley, Merthyr Tydfil and the other towns at the heads of the Valleys to the M50 at Ross. Between these two east-west arteries there are a few branch railway lines and only one fast road, that between Cardiff and Merthyr Tydfil. In the early 1990s there were few other fast roads serving the Valleys (although some are now being built), and so most of the population have good reason to feel isolated and cut off. Travel for both patients and health workers is difficult. Roads are poor and frequently busy. Public transport is irregular and expensive. What this implies for the organisation of PHC is a high rate of home visits, frequent use of branch surgeries, and a general problem in providing easy access to health care for those most in need.

In our experience, a sense of isolation characterises many of those working in PHC in the area. Moreover, health service colleagues who are based in Cardiff similarly think of the Valleys as being more distant than they actually are. The various departments in the College of Medicine that are involved in PHC have much more to do with PHCTs in Cardiff and the coastal area than with those in the Valleys. A good illustration of this perspective came in a TCV meeting when the location of the 1993 Conference was being planned. One view was that it was critical that it should be held in a new hotel in the Rhondda, well within the area. Those we had worked with, it was argued, would then feel that the conference was being held in their territory. The other view was that it should be held in Cardiff: how, it was asked, would the 'important' people know how to get to the Rhondda?

Illness and deprivation

The Valleys have a long history of illness and deprivation, largely arising out of industrialisation and the demands that this places upon manual workers and their families (Hart, 1971; Humphrys, 1972; Williams, 1985; Harris, 1987). The ways in which the economy of the area was adjusting to the collapse of the deep-mining industry and related industrial change during the late 1980s and early 1990s, is well reviewed by Rutherford (1991). The statistics on the levels of illness and disability in the area were well-known to the Welsh Office and so it had no difficulty in incorporating a health element into the Valleys Initiative.

The statistics on long-standing illness are perhaps the most important for PHC, directly representing as they do pressure upon PHCTs. The 1991 Census was the first national census to inquire into this aspect of health, the key question having been developed and tested through the national General Household Survey: 'Does the person have any long-term illness, health problem or handicap which limits his/her daily activities or the work he/she can do?'. The contrast in health between South Wales and the rest of Britain that this reveals could hardly be more striking. The eight areas with the highest rates of long-standing illness in the whole of Britain are all found in South Wales in the TCV area (County Statistics, 1991 Census for England and Wales, Table E).

This Census statistic, limiting long-standing illness, reflects of course perceived health status rather than clinically assessed health. But, as such, it directly represents the demand that is placed upon PHC services. Moreover, despite some sociologically interesting discrepancies, subjective indicators of ill-health are strongly correlated with clinically assessed illness. More generally, most indicators of illness and of the need for health care are highly inter-correlated at the geographical level:

> 'Wards with high mortality are likely to be wards with high levels of chronic sickness and disability, and a higher than average incidence of low birth weights – and vice versa in localities with good health records. This is not to pretend that there are no wards that defy such characterisation – most of them, it must be said, in rural areas. Yet patterns of ill-health are by and large cumulative: different kinds of health advantage or health burden tend to reinforce one another...'
> (Phillimore and Beattie, 1994: 66).

This argument implies that when a 100% census indicates that the South Wales Valleys have levels of self-assessed long-standing illness that are conspicuously the highest in the whole country, then this also indicates that it will be amongst the highest on many other indicators of ill-health and deprivation. The reasons for high levels in South Wales should of course be subject to detailed research (Lyons *et al.*, 1995). Undoubtedly the reasons would include some reference to the distinctive culture of South Wales in which disability and illness and regular absence from physically demanding work are intimately connected, and in which the health service has a heavy involvement in the regulation of employment and welfare benefits. But the main reason, of course, is the health-damaging environment of the post-war era in which occupational hazards and environmental pollution have constantly lowered the health of the local population.

The response of the health service

> 'In areas of most sickness and death, general practitioners have more work, larger lists, less hospital support and inherit more clinically ineffective traditions of consultation, than in the healthiest areas; ... the availability of good medical care tends to vary inversely with the need of the population served.' (Hart, 1971:405)

Implicit in Hart's Inverse Care Law is the idea that areas of high need are deprived of good medical care. Efforts have been made over recent years to develop ways of measuring high need or deprivation, and thus demand for health care services, to enable the distribution of extra resources to such areas. Deprivation is a key concept in regard to health service policy (Jarman, 1983). Mid Glamorgan Health Authority, for example, undertook a comprehensive analysis of the health of the county's population in 1985 and concluded that the population of Mid Glamorgan:

> '...suffers disproportionate levels of illness and disability and at the same time suffers high levels of adverse social conditions greater than other areas in Wales and England' (Mid Glamorgan HA, 1985).

A new system of payments to GPs was introduced with the new GP Contract in April 1990. This amounted to a capitation supplement for each patient living in a ward that scored 30 or more on the Jarman index of deprivation (Jarman, 1983; Lorentzon *et al.*, 1994). The index had been designed originally to reflect increases in GP workload and was based upon the following eight measures:

- % elderly living alone
- % under fives
- % unskilled
- % households overcrowded
- % single parent households
- % residents in ethnic minority households
- % unemployed
- % moved house.

Jarman's index was immediately subjected to critical analysis. Perhaps the most formidable challenge came from Townsend *et al.* (1987), and their alternative index has subsequently been used by many authorities, including Mid Glamorgan and Gwent Health Authorities, to advocate a more equitable distribution of payments (Hutchinson *et al.*, 1989). This index is based on indicators of unemployment, overcrowding, non-car ownership and non-owner occupation.

The inadequacy of the Jarman index was clearly apparent when applied to Wales. It generated average scores which indicated that the four least deprived counties in Wales were Mid and West Glamorgan, Dyfed and Powys. It was recognised by the government that, with the

Valleys appearing to be one of the least deprived parts of Wales, the Jarman index was an unsatisfactory indicator of deprivation in the Principality. To overcome this failure, the Welsh Office modified the Jarman index by incorporating standardised mortality ratios and statistics from the Welsh Office Housing Condition Survey. It was on the basis of this index that payments were made to GPs in Wales in the early 1990s. This ensured that deprivation payments, based upon this index, were concentrated in the Valleys. Of a total of 806 electoral wards in Wales, 52 were identified as deprived and warranting payments and of these 34 (65%) were in the TCV area. There was, however, considerable variation and even in the Valleys the majority of wards (77%) carried no payments. The consequence of this, as we discovered, was considerable dissatisfaction when one practice could be receiving several thousand pounds each year in deprivation payments and a neighbouring practice, serving what appeared to be a similar population, receiving no payments.

What this issue exemplifies is the complicated challenge that meeting the needs of areas of deprivation presents to health service policy. Investment by the Welsh Office in TCV is another example of extra expenditure being targeted on a distinctive geographical area as a result of proven deprivation. By launching the Programme for the Valleys, the Welsh Office was indicating that the government accepted the principle of targeting areas defined by census statistics and not by NHS administrative boundaries.

Teamcare Valleys

The following extract from the 1988 document setting out the Valleys Initiative describes the original rationale for establishing TCV:

'The Welsh Office will take a number of new initiatives designed to support the development of primary health care services for Valleys communities. The intention will be to extend vocational training for health professionals working in the Valleys and to provide a more direct role for the University of Wales College of Medicine. Measures to support improved team work in the primary care field will also be devised. These initiatives will be discussed with a range of interests, including the relevant Family Practitioner Committees, District Health Authorities, professional organisations and the College of Medicine itself. The aim will be to focus on service provision to achieve the best possible effect in the use of primary health care resources for the Valleys.' (Welsh Office, 1988:31)

This statement provides a clear indication of the rather nebulous nature of the expectations that arose from the initial agreement between the Welsh Office and the College of Medicine. There was a lack of definition which, while enabling flexibility in the development of a more detailed strategy for TCV, also contributed to divergent expectations between stakeholders and to some confusion among those required to develop that strategy.

Following the decision in 1988 it was not until 1990 that TCV was launched. 1990 was also a period of significant upheaval in the NHS with the introduction of the new Contract for GPs and the development of hospital and community trusts. 1990 was a significant year for PHC development but perhaps not the most propitious year to launch a new project.

Institutionally TCV was established as a multidisciplinary unit of the University of Wales College of Medicine linked to the Department of General Practice, the Department of Postgraduate Medical and Dental Education and the School of Nursing Studies. The staff appointed to TCV were also appointed members of staff of one of the parent departments. For example the editors of this book were appointed Senior Lecturers in the School of Nursing Studies and the Department of General Practice, respectively.

Aims and organisation

The aims of TCV are outlined in the TCV Strategy Document issued in 1990:

'The overall aims of Teamcare Valleys are to:

(1) Make a significant contribution to the sponsorship of better health in the valleys as well as helping to develop treatment services.
(2) Provide support of direct operational value to assist the delivery of primary care in the valleys.
(3) Provide a source of professional, research, managerial and entrepreneurial expertise to place at the disposal of primary care practitioners in the valleys.
(4) Promote the positive benefits of multi and interdisciplinary team working in primary care (for the community and practitioners alike) through training and other practical measures.
(5) Aim to sustain and complement the commitment of all those involved in primary care throughout the area.' (Welsh Office, 1990:7)

Early on, the staff of TCV decided that a simpler statement of the overall aim of TCV was needed, and initially it was proposed that this should be: 'The purpose of Teamcare Valleys is to develop primary health care in the Valleys area'. Following discussion, however, it was agreed that the word 'help' should be added in order to emphasise that it was the PHCTs themselves who were responsible for, and should be credited with, developing PHC. The primary purpose of TCV was to be supportive rather than directive: 'to help develop primary health care in the Valleys area'.

The project was staffed by a team of people, recruited largely from within South Wales. In all, 53 people were employed in TCV during the three years of the project (see Appendix 1). Over half, 37, were appointed as 'clinical fellows': experienced PHC practitioners, mostly coming from practice in the Valleys and appointed to undertake a wide range of projects. They were drawn from general practice, district nursing, health visiting, community psychiatric nursing, health promotion and midwifery, and were employed either full- or part-time, either as long-term (i.e. three year) clinical fellows, or as short-term clinical fellows for one or more sessions a week for a period from a few months up to two years.

The work of TCV was based on the broad aims described above but, in the concluding report summarizing the activities of the project, the Director, Dr Brian Wallace, identified three main themes which had underpinned activities:

- 'exploration of the concept of fellowships for primary health care practitioners;
- evaluation and promotion of the positive benefits of PHC teamworking;
- addressing the failure to disseminate and apply existing knowledge to patient care.' (TCV, 1993:1)

The work and activities of TCV developed in a number of directions which, for management purposes, were grouped under four headings:

- Field projects
- Practical support and advice
- Education and training programmes
- Communication.

The Field Projects were largely studies undertaken by the clinical fellows (and these contribute to the larger part of this book). As such, a clinical fellow was a project worker undertaking a project of relevance to the development of PHC in the Valleys area. But, at the same time, it was expected that most of the clinical fellows would continue in, or return to, PHC and so one objective was that they would acquire an understanding of, and experience in, the design and conduct of research and development projects. In our view this strategy for the development of PHC practitioners is sound but, in the context of a large and essentially short-term initiative such as TCV, it places considerable strains upon those who are appointed (see Chapters 10, 13, 15 and 18, for example).

Under Practical Support and Advice, TCV undertook activities that were focused on particular teams or individuals working in the Valleys who were trying to promote and develop their services. Advice was offered to PHCTs on the development of clinical practice and the management of general practice. Support was offered to a range of groups; for example, members of professional groups who are rather more isolated and vulnerable to stress and unreasonable workloads. Chapters 2 and 6 provide more detail about some of the activities of TCV in this area.

Education and Training encompassed a range of activities: educational needs assessment, the provision of courses, the development of distance learning courses, and the evaluation of educational activities. Some of these courses provided by TCV were aimed at one professional group, for example GPs (as discussed in Chapter 12) or practice managers (see Chapter 3). Other courses were aimed at the whole PHCT. One significant example of this, in which TCV made a substantial investment, was the tutor-facilitated distance learning course 'Community and Public Health in the Valleys' (Slater, 1993). This is a 25 week course that examines the effects of poverty and inequalities on health, and on the perceptions and work of those involved in providing PHC. A total of 34 students enrolled when this course was launched. They included district nurses, GPs, practice nurses, health visitors, specialist nurses, CHC representatives, and FHSA personnel.

Communication activities included the compilation and distribution of a quarterly newsletter, *ReValley*. A total of 3500 copies of each issue were distributed. Wherever possible, copies of *ReValley* were delivered to health centres and practice premises in person. This helped us maintain contact with many of the practices and provided opportunities for obtaining information and contributions for future editions. The size of *ReValley* expanded over the three years from four to sixteen pages and, as well as covering all of TCV activities, it attracted many contributions from practitioners in the area.

A series of four roadshows were held in 1991 and again in 1992 at different locations covering the area. These roadshows enabled local PHCTs to learn of each other's work and projects as well as providing TCV with an additional method of undertaking needs assessment (see Chapter 12), and of informing people in the area of our activities. They created opportunities for contact and exchange in parts of the TCV area that rarely hosted such gatherings.

Perhaps the most important activity under Communication was the organisation of the conference 'Changing Primary Health Care', held in the Rhondda in 1993 towards the end of the three year life of TCV. This brought together many people involved in PHC throughout the area, and attracted practitioners, managers and researchers in PHC from many parts of Britain and from as far afield as Australia (Parsons, 1993a). Project reports were distributed widely at the conference and this formed an additional opportunity to disseminate the findings and recommendations arising from the wide range of TCV activities.

A Steering Group was set up to oversee the activities of TCV and this included representatives of the University, local health authorities, FHSAs and the Welsh Office. Later this group became reconstituted as the Strategy Group and a smaller Programme Board was set up to oversee the work of TCV on behalf of the Welsh Office. Dr Peter Elwood, Director of the Medical Research Council Epidemiology Unit, was chair of the Steering Group and then of the Strategy Group.

Challenges

At the outset, the staff of TCV had to face a number of challenges including the establishment of:

- a staff team that understood and was committed to good team-working practices;
- a coherent system of working within the confined space of four Portakabins – this meant shared space and resources, developing good teamwork and reaching agreement over group objectives;
- communication channels and working relationships with a large number of PHC practitioners in the area who were keen to be involved – we estimated that about 3000 people were contracted or employed to provide PHC in the Valleys and we wanted to involve as many as possible in TCV activities;
- links with DHAs, FHSAs and educational providers in the area – this was a real challenge given their statutory responsibilities, their own concerns about resources and their predictable and understandable suspicion of an initiative that threatened to complicate their own developmental work;
- links and joint activities with parent academic departments;
- a shared understanding with the Steering Group of the work implicit in the aims and objectives of TCV.

These challenges involved many different groups of people, who had very different expectations of TCV and were looking for different types of outcome. For example, some health service managers were concerned with the contribution that TCV could make towards achieving government targets, while PHC practitioners were much more concerned with resource needs and with day-to-day interpersonal relationships in their teams (which had to be addressed before attention could be focused on wider targets). Academic departments on the other hand were concerned about their academic ratings and about the development of members of staff in terms of the quality of their research.

The pulls of these different demands were often difficult to resolve (see, for example, Chapters 7, 9, 10, 15 and 17). One of the main lessons we learnt from the TCV experience is the need for all stakeholders to be explicit about their expectations, to acknowledge the legitimacy of the expectations of others, and for them to reach some consensus about identifying realistic objectives for the project as a whole. It is also necessary for project teams to carefully assess their ability to meet demands and expectations, particularly where demands are competing for the resources, time and expertise of the staff of the project.

The aim of this book

Our aim in preparing this book for publication has been to provide a record of some of the activities that were undertaken in the name of TCV. Lessons can be drawn from these accounts by others involved in, or embarking upon, PHC development activities. The aim in each chapter has been not only to provide an account of individual projects, the activities that were undertaken and the wider lessons that can be learnt, but also to provide an idea of what is involved in this kind of development work. Any number of projects could have been drawn upon for inclusion in this collection and those that are included demonstrate the diversity of activities that made up TCV. Unlike some PHC development projects, TCV was multi-faceted and multi-layered and addressed the issues of PHC development from all angles rather than through a single approach. A peculiar feature of TCV is that it did not claim ownership of many of the projects in which it was actively involved. While this degree of complexity and ambiguity was at times difficult for those outside to comprehend and evaluate, for the practices and PHC practitioners with whom we collaborated, it appeared to make a great deal of sense (see, for example, Chapters 2, 8, 16, 20 and 22). PHC is of itself complex and multi-layered and we consider that a multifaceted approach such as that tested by TCV has considerable potential in achieving real change.

The book is organised in five sections which reflect the activities of TCV and the concerns of PHC in the early 1990s: Management, Audit, Education, Community Needs and Teamwork. While each of the sections focuses on a particular area of TCV work all the chapters are based on the aims of TCV and thus illustrate individually and collectively how TCV sought to help develop PHC in the Valleys. Each section may be considered on its own by those who are interested in one topic rather than another but within the different sections there are considerable interconnections. For example, Chapter 6 focuses on the needs of different professional groups and has links with the Teamwork Section, and Chapter 16 describes a project which grew out of audit activities and thus has links to Section 2. Each section has a brief introduction in which we outline the more prominent themes in the chapters that follow.

In this first chapter we have aimed to introduce TCV and place the work of TCV and the PHC practitioners in the Valleys in the wider context. We learnt from the Rhondda conference that many features of our experience we share with projects working in similarly deprived or challenging locations, such as those in inner cities or rural areas (Parsons, 1993b; Pringle, 1993; Ealing, Hammersmith and Hounslow Health Agency, 1994; Thomas, 1995). Indeed we would argue that the South Wales Valleys have one particular feature in common with most other areas: the remarkable dedication of most PHCTs and their will-ingness to learn and adapt when faced with the challenges of change. Dr Peter Elwood, Chairman of the Steering Committee, was able to conclude at the end of the project:

> 'In its short life TCV clearly demonstrated something of the potential benefits of a unit which spanned academic departments of the Col-lege of Medicine and primary health care workers, and which, by working alongside the primary health care teams, and by involving the primary care workers themselves, sought the application of new knowledge and not just the collection of data. ... As a pilot scheme it had a remarkable success ... the spin-off and the ongoing effects of this highly imaginative enterprise will undoubtedly be consider-able.' (TCV, 1993: Foreword)

The lessons being learnt about PHC development are gradual and incremental and it is our hope that this book will provide another piece of the jigsaw and add to the ongoing effects of TCV. In this context, it seems appropriate to end this chapter with the words of the Welsh poet Dylan Thomas:

> 'I have heard many years of telling,
> And many years should see some change.

> The ball I threw while playing in the park
> Has not yet reached the ground.'
> (From *Should lanterns shine*, Jones, 1971: 116. Extract from *Dylan Thomas. The Poems*, published by J.M. Dent, London and New Directions Publishing Corporation, New York. Reproduced with permission.)

References

Bosanquet, N. (1995) Reviving the sleeping beauty. *Health Service Journal*, **105**(5448), 20–22.

Bryar, R. (1994a) *Nursing Outcomes of Teamcare Valleys 1990–1993*. Welsh Office, Cardiff.

Bryar, R. (1994b) An examination of the need for new nursing roles in primary health care. *Journal of Interprofessional Care*, **8**(1), 73–84.

Bytheway, B. (1991) *Primary Health Care Needs*. TCV Discussion Paper 8. TCV, Welsh Office, Cardiff.

Ealing, Hammersmith and Hounslow Health Agency (1994) *Primary Health Care Education Centre Evaluation Strategy.* Ealing, Hammersmith and Hounslow Health Agency, London.

Harris, C.C. (1987) *Redundancy and Recession in South Wales.* Basil Blackwell, Oxford.

Hart, J.T. (1971) The inverse care law. *The Lancet,* **i**, 405–412.

Humphrys, G. (1972) *Industrial Britain: Industrial South Wales.* David and Charles, Newton Abbott.

Hutchinson, A., Foy, C. & Sandhu, B. (1989) Comparison of two scores for allocating resources to doctors in deprived areas. *British Medical Journal,* **299**, 1142–4.

Jarman, B. (1983) Identification of underprivileged areas. *British Medical Journal,* **286**, 1705–8.

Jenkins, R. & Edwards, A. (eds) (1990) *One Step Forward? South and West Wales Towards the Year 2000.* Social Science Research Institute, Swansea, and Gorner Press, Llandysul.

Jones, D. (1971) *Dylan Thomas. The Poems.* Dent, London.

Lorentzon, M., Jarman, B. & Bajekal, M. (1994) *Report of the Inner City Task Force of the Royal College of General Practitioners.* Occasional Paper 66. The Royal College of General Practitioners, London.

Lyons, R.A., Fielder, H. & Littlepage, B.N.C. (1995) Measuring health status with the SF-36: the need for regional norms. *Journal of Public Health Medicine,* **17**(1), 46–50.

Mid Glamorgan Health Authority (1985) *Deprivation and Health.* Mid Glamorgan Health Authority, Cardiff.

NHSE (1994) *Developing NHS Purchasing and GP Fundholding Towards a Primary Care-led NHS.* NHSE, DoH, Leeds.

Owens, P., Carrier, J. & Horder, J. (Eds) (1995) *Interprofessional Issues in Community and Primary Health Care.* Macmillan, London.

Parsons, S. (1993a) *Conference '93: Final Report.* TCV, Welsh Office, Cardiff.

Parsons, S. (ed) (1993b) *Changing Primary Health Care.* A collection of papers from the Teamcare Valleys Conference 1993. TCV, Welsh Office, Cardiff.

Pearson, P. & Spencer, J. (in press) *Promoting Teamwork in Primary Care: A Research Based Approach.* Arnold, London.

Pendleton, D. (1995) Professional development in general practice: problems, puzzles and paradigms. *British Journal of General Practice,* **45**, 377–81.

Phillimore, P. & Beattie, A. (1994) *Health and Inequality in the Northern Region 1981–1991. A Report.* Department of Social Policy, University of Newcastle, Newcastle-upon-Tyne.

Pringle, M. (1993) *Change and Teamwork in Primary Care.* BMJ Publishing Group, London.

Review of Community Nursing in Wales (1987) *Nursing in the Community – A Team Approach for Wales.* Welsh Office, Cardiff.

Rutherford, T. (1991) Industrial restructuring, local labour markets and social change: the transformation of South Wales. In: *Contemporary Wales* (eds G. Day and G. Rees), **4**, 9–44. University of Wales Press, Cardiff.

Secretary of State for Health (1989) *Working for Patients.* HMSO, London.

Slater, J. (1993) *Community and Public Health in the Valleys.* A Teamcare Valleys Multi-disciplinary Distance Learning Course, October 1992 to June 1993. Evaluation Report. TCV, Welsh Office, Cardiff.

Standing Nursing and Midwifery Advisory Committee (1995) *Making it happen. Public Health – the Contribution, Role and Development of Nurses, Midwives and Health Visitors.* DoH, London.

Tarimo, E. & Webster, E.G. (1994) *Primary Health Care Concepts and Challenges in a Changing World. Alma-Ata Revisited.* SHS Paper number 7. Division of Strengthening of Health Services, World Health Organization, Geneva.

TCV (1993) *University of Wales College of Medicine Teamcare Valleys 1990–1993. Overview Report.* TCV, Welsh Office, Cardiff.

Thomas, P. (1995) There is hope yet for the development of primary health care in deprived areas. *British Journal of General Practice,* **45,** 572–4.

Tollman, S. (1991) Community oriented primary care: origins, evolution, applications. *Social Science and Medicine,* **32**(6), 633–42.

Townsend, P., Phillimore, P. & Beattie, A. (1987) *Health and Deprivation: Inequality and the North.* Croom Helm, Beckenham.

Vetter, N. (1995) *The Hospital. From Centre of Excellence to Community Support.* Chapman & Hall, London.

Wallace, B. (1993) The Teamcare Valleys Initiative. *Health and Social Care in the Community,* **1**(1), 61–4.

Welsh Office (1988) *The Valleys. A Programme for the People.* Welsh Office, Cardiff.

Welsh Office (1990) *Teamcare Valleys Strategy.* TCV, Welsh Office, Cardiff.

West, M. (1994) *Effective Teamwork.* The British Psychological Society, Leicester.

Williams, G. (1985) *When was Wales? A History of the Welsh.* Penguin, Harmondsworth.

Wilson, A. (1994) *Changing Practices in Primary Care. A Facilitator's Handbook.* Health Education Authority, London.

WHO (1988) *From Alma-Ata to the Year 2000. Reflections at the Midpoint.* WHO, Geneva.

WHO (1994) *Nursing beyond the Year 2000.* Report of a WHO Study Group. WHO Technical Report Series 842. WHO, Geneva.

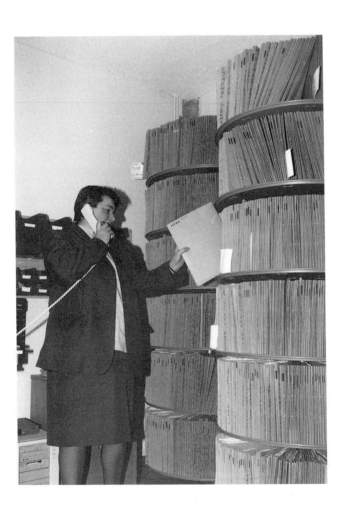

Section 1

Management

The introduction of the 1990 General Practitioner Contract, together with the enhanced role of Family Health Services Authorities (FHSAs), placed the spotlight on the management of PHC, an area which had traditionally received little attention. The chapters in this section consider ways in which the management of PHC may be developed, both through attention to issues directly relevant to the management of practices, and to issues which impact on management, such as individual behaviours and support mechanisms available to professional groups.

Day-to-day problems often experienced by practices include poor record systems, staff shortages and a growing workload. These problems may mask more deep-rooted problems of communication within the practice, financial issues or long-standing educational needs of team members. These problems may be resolved internally or practitioners may seek assistance from outside agencies. Chapter 2 reports upon the TCV experience of offering a multi-disciplinary advice and support service to practices. Three common problems experienced by the practices with whom the service was involved were identified: appointing staff, managing workload and troubleshooting. In addition, individual practices presented a range of needs, some of which were met internally via TCV's educational and other resources and some were met by other agencies.

Chapter 3 focuses on the present state of management in practices: what are the educational requirements of practice managers and other support staff? What are the implications of current policy developments for managers and receptionists? What should be the priorities of health purchasers in the provision of training opportunities? In this chapter an outline is given of the policy changes which have had such a significant impact on the role of management in PHC. Initiatives in developing management education in practices are described. This chapter illustrates both TCV's work in seeking to meet the needs of one group of PHC practitioners and demonstrates the ways in which TCV worked with other local organisations to meet identified needs. The basis of this chapter is the view that high quality practice management is essential for high quality PHC and that there is considerable work still to be done in developing career structures and education in PHC management.

A particular responsibility in practice management is to health and safety. All employers have certain statutory responsibilities under Health and Safety legislation. This has recently been extended to cover the premises of health services. The health service should be particularly sensitive to the importance of this since failures inevitably lead to increased demands upon its own limited resources. How aware are those involved in the provision of PHC services of their responsibilities? What is the level of knowledge and compliance with Health and Safety requirements? Chapter 4 investigates what practice managers can do to ensure high levels of health and safety in the surgery and health centre.

The final two chapters in this section focus on the needs of individuals within the practice team. Chapter 5 is the report of a survey of GPs in the TCV area, enquiring into their health, health-related behaviour and the pressure they felt from their work. This study was undertaken by two GPs who held short-term clinical fellowships with TCV. The surprising findings of this study challenge the received wisdom about GPs' health behaviours and would benefit from replication on a wider scale. It suggests that GPs, on the whole, do adjust their habits – smoking, drinking and exercise – in order to maintain good health. There is also some evidence that the health of those doctors with heavy workloads may suffer as a consequence. It is argued that the answer may rest partly in better time management. The relationship that is demonstrated between good time management and health related behaviour is something which could be addressed in GP vocational training and in continuing medical education activities.

While one aim of TCV was to develop multidisciplinary teamworking, individuals also need support and interaction with members of their own professional groups. Some members of the PHCT tend to be isolated from other members of their own professional group for a variety of reasons. In order to complement multidisciplinary teamwork, many value the opportunity to share ideas and anxieties with others in comparable positions in other localities, and thereby to extend their knowledge and skills. Chapter 6 compares the organisation and activities of support or self-help groups for nurse educators, practice managers and solo general practitioners.

These chapters focus primarily upon the management of the practice and its relations with regulatory and support agencies and other stakeholders in the health service. All raise questions about how practices can have access to support as they develop and adjust to the challenges of changing national policies and regulations.

A key lesson that comes out of this section is how the autonomy of the PHC professional and isolation of the PHCT can generate major challenges to the management of service delivery. There is a useful role for agencies such as TCV which, through advice and education, can help groups find solutions to what may seem like insuperable problems.

Chapter 2

Helping to Resolve Problems in the Development of Practices

Brian Wallace

There are major changes currently taking place in PHC as a consequence of changing demography, disease patterns and concepts of health, advances in health care, and government policy to shift resources out of hospitals into the community. The challenges facing those working in the PHC sector include:

- an expanding, changing role – which will require them to review their professional responsibilities as well as to acquire new knowledge and skills;
- multidisciplinary work – increasingly health care will be provided by teams (which are likely to include new disciplines), as the effective use of resources to produce health gains demands a multidisciplinary approach to patient care;
- the application of new knowledge and skills in practice, and
- improving standards of care – through the establishment of widespread professional audit procedures.

Implementing change in practice

The continuity between research, development and practice has been recognised to be fundamental to developing a knowledge-driven health service (Welsh Office, 1992). However, Hart (1988), amongst others, has commented on the lack of use of research in medical science and general practice, and it has been argued that, more important than establishing a framework for research and development, is doing something about the failure to disseminate and apply existing knowledge (Editorial, 1991).

Luker (1993), in investigating the diffusion of innovations in PHC, found that their adoption was delayed by the organisational and financial constraints of working within a small practice. Adoption could be speeded up if positive support and inducements were available to practices. These findings are very much in keeping with experience of the diffusion of technological innovations in commercial companies (Coombs *et al.*, 1987). For example, the Enterprise Initiative of the Department of Trade and Industry is a consultancy scheme providing advice, guidance and practical help to small or medium-size businesses without: 'the time for proper analysis and planned development' (Department of Trade and Industry, 1991:1). The intention is to help such businesses become more successful by providing access to outside professional advisers.

Leese and Bosanquet (1995:705), following a survey of the effects of recent changes in general practice strategy, concluded that: 'the new range of incentives has proved powerful and effective in securing change ... (but) differences remained, depending on the location and philosophy of the practice'. Haines and Jones (1994), in considering methods of encouraging the implementation of the findings of research, note the limitations of a 'top down' approach and of formal education. To counter this, Harris (1993:190) anticipated that:

> 'exciting possibilities exist for collaboration (of FHSAs) with academic departments of general practice and other primary care disciplines, such as attachments, exchanges and joint research projects and the joint formulation of independent service research units, fostering research and development on multi-disciplinary team work and integrated care'.

The case for such collaboration involving the active participation of all members of the PHCT was confirmed by the experience of TCV (see Chapters 7, 8, 14 and 21, for example). Educational and training programmes, with the emphasis upon multi-disciplinary learning, were devised to meet identified needs in the TCV area. These were shown to produce measurable changes in knowledge, but were not sufficient to lead to early changes in professional behaviour and practice organisation.

The Practice Advisory Service

The overall aims of TCV included the provision of support of direct operational value to PHC in the Valleys, and to place at the disposal of practices a source of professional, research, managerial and entrepreneurial expertise (TCV, 1990). To this end the Practice Advisory Service was established with the aim of supporting practices involved in changing the way they were organised and managed. The expertise and experience of the senior staff of TCV were drawn together to offer this service. The core team was myself, Stephanie Williams and Rosamund Bryar, with backgrounds in medicine, management and nursing, respectively. Other members of TCV staff were asked to visit practices when there was a need for assistance relevant to their expertise. The objectives were to help practices identify problems and generate solutions through an assessment of their organisation, their services, and their staff and patient needs, and by advising them upon these aspects of their practice.

It was planned that the Service would be limited to a diagnostic and advisory function, to avoid duplicating the responsibilities of other agencies. Some practices, however, expected much more:

- funding for staffing, equipment or building;
- additional service staff;
- instant solutions rather than help in learning how to identify and solve current and future problems themselves.

The availability of TCV staff time proved to be a major constraint – the core team met as a management group approximately once every two months and could only assist a maximum of six practices at any one time.

Procedure

The advisory procedure involved a number of steps in helping a practice. Initially the practice was asked to complete a structured questionnaire intended to produce systematic information about practice staffing and function. Often there was a poor response to this request. Some practices seemed to be suspicious of providing detailed practice information in print – they preferred to talk face-to-face.

Following this initial contact, two or three core team members visited the practice to meet the people working there, to discuss the issues raised and to identify the nature of the difficulties to be addressed. If involvement of the Service appeared to be appropriate, an action plan was agreed with the people concerned. If, on the other hand, involvement seemed to be inappropriate, the practice was advised to seek the help of other agencies.

It was often necessary for a practice to obtain detailed data concerning the aspect of its work that was presenting problems. In this situation, TCV designed data recording sheets specifically for the needs of the particular practice. With these it was possible to perform brief audits of, for example: GPs' and practice nurses' workload, age and sex distribution of patients seen, patients called for review, and prescribing patterns.

Although the source of information was usually systems already established in the practice, appointment books or surgery lists, for example, the transfer of information was perceived as 'extra work' by practice staff. It was important to ensure that the effort involved was less than the subsequent return. The information provided was then analysed and used to help the practice make decisions about the changes required to solve the problems presented. Supportive contact was maintained with the practice during implementation of the action plan. Progress was reviewed periodically in order to assess progress and evaluate the effect of the intervention by the Service.

Of problems that were presented by practices, 40% were associated with appointing new staff, 30% concerned workload and 30% involved 'troubleshooting'.

Appointing new staff

All the problems practices had in appointing new staff arose from the changes brought in by the 1990 GP Contract with the NHS. An increased awareness of the possible benefits of additional staff, the changing role of practice managers and nurses, and the availability of pump-priming funding, combined to expose weaknesses in personnel management. This applied to the larger, more sophisticated, practices as well as to the smaller, more traditional, ones (see Chapter 3).

All the tasks of appointing new staff were satisfactorily completed over an average period of three months, involving an average of four contacts between the practice and the Advisory Service. One intervention was very rushed, help being sought late in the process of appointing a manager when it was realised by the practice that mistakes had already been made. Another intervention developed slowly over eight months as other changes were taking place in the practice.

The issues that practices encounter in appointing people to management positions include:

- Appointing people from within practices and changing their responsibilities. For example, a receptionist may be appointed as practice manager, or a practice manager become a fund-holding manager. Problems arise if these people do not want to change, preferring, for example, patient contact to working in an office, or doubting their own capability to take on additional responsibilities. The employing practitioners may have encouraged such people to 'try it' and then become disappointed with an apparent failure to take on the expanded role.
- Detailing or clarifying the anticipated responsibilities of a post. Some of these responsibilities may not have existed before in the practice.
- Finding, short-listing and interviewing people. In some practices, the partners may have no experience of the appointment process.
- Establishing procedures for replacing staff. As the complexity and workload of a practice increases, so does the importance of teamwork. To minimise the damage of unexpected resignations, it is

necessary to have efficient procedures for filling vacancies as quickly as possible.

Despite the rapid increase in the number of practice nurses and changes in their role, few problems were presented to the Advisory Service regarding their appointment. It may be that general practitioners felt more confident in handling clinical appointments, though evidence of the suitability of some of those made is not reassuring (see Chapter 11). The problems that were presented raised issues similar to those of appointing practice managers:

- definition of role in relationship to the needs of the practice;
- replacing staff who could not cope with the increasing responsibilities;
- selection procedures;
- training staff in post to assume new responsibilities.

The demand for outside help with staff appointments was largely precipitated by changes in NHS regulations, although it can be anticipated that there will be a continuing need for help in this area as practices develop. This need could well be met by an NHS agency as long as it is able to provide a sensitive personal service.

Workload

Problems in coping with workload were more often raised in practices where contact with TCV had been established for some other reason – a variation on the 'while you're here, Doctor' syndrome! In some of these practices, the initial interview identified a single, comparatively simple problem. In others the presented problem was discovered to be just part of a larger difficulty (see Chapter 5).

The complaint 'The morning surgeries just go on and on and on!' led to a workload analysis in one well-established three-partner practice. This was conducted under the supervision of the practice manager over a two-week period. This covered the complete cycle of surgeries and clinics. It showed a workload equivalent to 4.5 contacts per patient per year – higher than the national, but lower than the local, average. Numbers of house calls were low but the 10 minute surgery appointments often went on for longer. The problem for this caring practice was that it did not have sufficient spaces in the appointments book to accommodate the consultations it provided in practice.

Subsequently we considered the question: why couldn't this practice solve this problem internally? At the initial interview, no one was aware of the patient consultation rate, the doctors' average consultation times, or the distribution of consultations during the week. Hopefully, with increased management skills, practice problems such as these will be routinely anticipated and resolved in the future.

The claim 'We haven't got enough time to cope, let alone start new things!' was the introduction to a series of problems in a two-partner practice set in a particularly deprived area. Analysis over one month confirmed that their workload was almost twice the national average. Over 50% of consultations concerned children under five years of age, and one partner asked 40% of patients seen to make a follow-up appointment. Sharing this information with the practice revealed a number of related problems: strained relationships with local health visitors, limited local parental confidence in handling minor illnesses in children, past experiences affecting the current practice of one of the doctors, and the practice manager being unhappy in her job. The practice was assisted in developing an action plan and in putting this into practice. This included a meeting with local health visitors, a parent education programme, and a review of the various responsibilities of practice staff.

Contact with this practice continued over ten months and involved sixteen sessions with the Service. This was a dysfunctional practice where the presenting problem of workload was an indication of more widespread problems. These required medical, nursing and management input, and sensitive support for the individuals involved. This kind of situation requires external help from experienced individuals from outside the NHS management system.

Troubleshooting

In relation to one third of the problems presented to the Service, the help of TCV was sought by an FHSA or MAAG that was concerned about a practice that was having difficulties. One FHSA identified a group of six practices which had failed to achieve immunisation and cytology targets. It invited TCV to help these practices to develop a strategy to achieve them. This challenge became a separate TCV project (Williams, 1993).

One of these six practices was found to require assistance in developing administrative systems and in specifying the role of the practice nurse. In another practice the initial interview revealed a worrying situation. Despite the efforts of the Service, this was not amenable to change until action was taken by the FHSA. In general there was slow progress with practices in this group due to a number of factors:

- The relationship between the TCV Service and the FHSA had to be clarified. Some practices viewed the FHSA with suspicion and, in these situations, it was more difficult for TCV to maintain its independence.
- Sufficient time was not available. The Service was only one part of the many activities of TCV.
- Once started, impetus had to be maintained. Many of these practices needed a person to be placed in the practice to bring about the changes required.

- Practices had unrealistic expectations of what TCV could do for them.
- Similarly, NHS management had unrealistic expectations that major changes could be achieved in a very short time.

The lessons learned

Although most of the problems and difficulties encountered by practices are resolved internally, sometimes there is a need for a source of external guidance or expertise. This is particularly so when PHCTs need help to translate newly gained theory or changed regulations into practice. This often involves changing established structures and procedures. While health authorities (HAs) have a role in this area, they may be constrained both by their statutory and regulatory responsibilities, and by a lack of appropriate skills and experience. Such skills and experience could be provided by an independent agency such as TCV.

Our experience suggests that help over difficulties with staff appointments could – and preferably should – be provided by the NHS. Hopefully, the HAs will build up a bank of informed experience in this area. In contrast, the challenges of understanding and resolving workload difficulties are best met within the practice, with the help of independent support provided by individuals with experience in the field. Dysfunctional practices with organisational problems may well require attention from both health purchasers and an advisory service working in close co-operation. There is a small but significant proportion of poorly organised practices that require substantial help from an agency that works alongside, although independently of, the NHS, in providing an integrated input to the practice.

It is essential that an advisory service and its members are, and are perceived to be, independent of NHS management. While FHSAs employed professional facilitators to help practices, their targets were management outcomes rather than aspects of more immediate concern to the practitioners involved. Practices are understandably wary of allowing outsiders to become involved and knowledgeable in the functioning of their business, if this might have an effect on their funding and on the allocation of other resources to them (see Chapter 10). The location of the TCV Service and its members in the University of Wales College of Medicine enabled this independence to be widely recognised.

The complex nature of problems that involve medical, nursing, management and ancillary staff demands a multidisciplinary team. Only then is it possible to identify the full implications of presented difficulties, to understand the impact of possible solutions and to develop and implement integrated plans. A multidisciplinary advisory team will also ensure that effective communication is established with all the relevant members of the PHCT. The various members of the advisory service must have experience of working in PHC to establish credibility, links with others to provide supplementary advice, and back-up from an established institution such as a university.

The limitations of a directive 'top down' approach to problems in PHC is that, although it may enhance the service with more equipment, more staff or more clinics, this does not necessarily guarantee improved and sustained patient care outcomes. If a PHCT is to fully implement a change in professional behaviour that contributes to better patient care, it is essential that it enjoys a sense of ownership. This can only be achieved through the direct involvement of its members in the assessment, planning and evaluation of any development. Sometimes they have to learn how to do this themselves, as change can only be facilitated from outside the practice if there is sufficient internal capability.

All aspects of a problem require attention in order to achieve sustained success. Many of the complex problems of PHC make it necessary to work at different levels, in a stepwise approach and with considerable flexibility. This can require a major input of staff time, and progress may be delayed by various factors, not least the slow response of a practice which has to maintain a continuing and demanding patient care service.

Although PHC development may have a long-term mission, practices are more interested in the short to medium-term benefits and consequences of changes in their activities. It is essential to establish targets which are considered useful and achievable in order to effect real change in practice.

References

Coombs, R., Saviotti, P. & Walsh, D. (1987) *Economics and Technological Change.* Macmillan Education, London.

Department of Trade and Industry (1991) *Consultancy. Application and Guidance.* HMSO, London.

Editorial (1991) Not R & D but DNA. *Health Services Management Research,* **87**(6), 242.

Haines, A. & Jones, R. (1994) Implementing findings of research. *British Medical Journal,* **308**, 1488–92.

Harris, A. (1993) Developing a research and development strategy for primary care. *British Medical Journal,* **306**, 189–92.

Hart, J.T. (1988) *A New Kind of Doctor.* Merlin Press, London.

Leese, B. & Bosanquet, N. (1995) Family doctors and change in practice strategies since 1988. *British Medical Journal,* **310**, 705–8.

Luker, K. (1993) Reflections on the diffusion of innovations in primary health care. In: *Changing Primary Health Care* (ed. S. Parsons). A collection of papers from the Teamcare Valleys Conference 1993, Chapter 1, 5–12. TCV, Welsh Office, Cardiff.

Teamcare Valleys (1990) *Strategy Document.* TCV, Welsh Office, Cardiff.

Welsh Office (1992) *Sharpening the Focus: Research and Development Framework for NHS Wales.* NHS Directorate, Welsh Office, Cardiff.

Williams, S. (1993) Making it Happen: Implementing Change in Practice. In: *Changing Primary Health Care* (ed. S. Parsons). A collection of papers from the Teamcare Valleys Conference 1993, Chapter 11, 52–5. TCV, Welsh Office, Cardiff.

Chapter 3

Developing Practice Management

Stephanie Williams

General practice, and the roles of practice managers within practices, have changed enormously since the introduction of the 1990 GP Contract. The Contract shifted the emphasis away from the management and treatment of disease towards the prevention of disease and health promotion. In support of this reorientation, practices were provided with incentive payments for vaccination and immunisation of pre-school children and for cervical cytology, and support was given to improve the range and quality of chronic disease management services. At the same time, the proportion of practice income that was based on capitation payments was reduced.

These changes have increased the range and importance of management tasks within practices. The range of tasks has shifted from purely administrative activities, such as making appointments and claiming from the FHSA for work carried out, to include many other management responsibilities. GPs and their teams now have to confront the resource consequences and opportunity costs that are implicit in the choices they make in deciding what services to offer, to which client group, when, where, and by whom.

Changes in responsibilities

During this same period, and in tandem with the changing emphasis on management at the practice level, the roles and responsibilities of the contracting agencies have also changed markedly. Prior to 1990, the Family Practitioner Committees (FPCs) existed mainly to ensure that the independent PHC contractors – GPs, dental practitioners, pharmacists and optometrists – carried out their contractual obligations and were appropriately reimbursed for so doing.

In 1990 FHSAs replaced the FPCs and, for the first time, the administrative agencies were to be responsible not just for the existence of primary care services, but also for their quality. These new agencies were headed up by General Managers who were appointed on short-term (three year) contracts. They were to be held personally accountable (with performance-related pay) for the achievement of the goals of their organisations. Their next contract was going to depend on their success in achieving these changes both within their own organisations and, even more importantly and more visibly, within the practices in their catchment area. These goals, set by the government, reflect the prevailing, and growing, public demand for tighter accountability within the professions, and for a greater responsiveness to consumer wishes.

The new emphasis on management also affected individual responsibilities at the local level. Practices rapidly discovered that the receptionist they had optimistically upgraded, and had previously regarded as a mine of information about practice systems, floundered and was, more often than not, overwhelmed by the new range of expectations placed upon her. Well-meaning GPs tried to help by picking up some of the management pieces, only to recoil in horror from the continuously growing burden, and the amount of time it took, taking them away from patient care. Not fully understanding the roles and functions of management themselves, they were often in no position to offer meaningful advice or support.

Many practice managers were in a peculiarly isolated position, both geographically and professionally. With no one in their practices to turn to, or to use as appropriate role models, and often with little experience of management functions outside of general practice, they were left to write their own rules. Consequently a widely divergent range of tasks came to be incorporated under the umbrella title of 'practice manager'. An equally variable range of pay and conditions were attached to the posts. Many GPs and practice managers lacked the skills to argue the case effectively for higher rates of pay and, with cash-limited budgets, it was not in the interests of the FHSAs to heed their pleas too hastily.

Current developments

Yet the roles and responsibilities of practice managers have continued to grow, and will continue to do so if the current policy drive to develop a PHC-led NHS is to be achieved. Current policy drives are bound to exacerbate these present trends. The increasing emphasis on treating patients as close as possible to their own homes and, where possible, in their homes, inevitably means that more demands will be placed on PHCTs.

Shorter lengths-of-stay, more day surgery, and the push to provide more consultant-led medical and therapeutic services outside the hospital, mean that hospital care will be reserved for the more acutely ill, admitted for shorter and shorter periods of time. PHCTs will be expected to provide a wider range of services to their patients, and perhaps to patients of neighbouring doctors as well. The drive to push responsibility for expenditure on patient care closer to the patient will mean additional responsibility for the GP and PHCTs; inevitably, Health Commissions will require increased accountability from GPs for expenditure committed. Practice managers will be required to set up the systems to implement this process.

In line with these changes, PHCTs will also grow in size, and increasingly the health and social care professionals who are attached to a practice will need clear definitions of their respective responsibilities, and careful co-ordination of their activities. Expenditure on health visitors and community nurses, as on social workers and community psychiatrist nurses, will have to be justified in terms of expected outcomes and improvements in the quality of care. Similarly practices will increasingly be required to attend to their legal duties regarding employment and the health and safety of those who work in their premises (see Chapter 4).

The professional most likely to have to bear the responsibility for co-ordinating these activities, for turning them into an effective team, and for proving that any expenditure committed is justified in terms of improved patient care, is likely to be the practice manager. Although improving quality is everyone's business, it is, by definition, only the manager in an organisation whose specific job role is 'to achieve the organisation's objectives and continuously improve its performance' (The Management Charter Initiative, 1991: 39). Working through other people, the manager will be responsible for ensuring that the organisation's resources, people, skills, premises, income, and time, are effectively deployed so that the most appropriate possible care is delivered to the right group of patients at the right time and in the right setting.

Developing educational opportunities for practice managers

When TCV was established the urgent task at hand regarding practice managers was the provision of appropriate development channels and support mechanisms. In this way practice managers would be helped to acquire the skills they needed to manage more effectively, both strategically and operationally, in this continually changing environment. What, we had to decide, were the essential elements to be included in that development process, and how could it best be organised and delivered? We recognised the problems arising from the distinctly isolated position of practice managers and took steps to help them establish a support group (see Chapter 6). In addition it was clear that education and training should be given a high priority.

Traditionally, management education and development has been provided through academic settings, and focused on the knowledge element of the learning triad: knowledge, attitudes and skills. Located in UWCM, TCV was well placed to follow in this tradition.

This approach, however, has been open to criticism on several fronts: knowledge, while arguably a necessary prerequisite, is not sufficient to ensure improved performance. We came to realise, in providing professional support and development work through TCV, that concentrating on improving knowledge sometimes has the opposite effect, that it serves to reinforce rather than to challenge existing attitudes and behaviours. Another problem with knowledge-based programmes is the difficulty of finding a common baseline from which to start. When working with practice managers, an emerging professional group whose responsibilities are so very varied, and whose qualifications and educational backgrounds are so different, there is both a remedial and a developmental challenge to be met. These challenges make structuring and delivering a programme appropriate to the needs of all the participants very difficult if not impossible.

Faced with these concerns, and charged in TCV with responsibility for creating innovative pathways in the development of practice management, I consulted Paul Hocking, then Development Officer for FHSAs in Wales. He had recognised similar problems in trying to provide appropriate and effective training opportunities. We decided we should experiment with competence-based approaches, and so set up a pilot NVQ5 project with practice managers in Gwent. This project, while successfully delivering the first NVQ5 practice managers' course in Wales (and possibly in the whole of the UK), also opened our eyes to the pitfalls of programmes based purely on standards of performance. Specific problems included:

- A lack of structure – although this was meant to suit participants in that they were 'free' to work at their own pace, in reality this often translated into 'no pace'.
- Individuals meant well and intended to make progress, but the work of compiling an NVQ portfolio always took second place to the operational demands of the workplace.
- The participants did not have to attend for teaching or instruction on a set day away from their workplace, and it was difficult for them to structure their time in work in a way that allowed them to follow the programme.
- The biggest problem with the competence approach, however, was the lack of any knowledge element. As 'occupationally competent' advisors, we were able to provide ad hoc teaching specific to the

needs of participants, but the cost implications of this were considerable.

In contrast, what we also learnt was that the main advantage of the competence-based approach was that it empowered the participants in enabling them to take control of their own professional development. This is singularly important with a group for whom appropriate professional role models are thin on the ground.

The 'Train the Trainers Programme'

Since 1990, FHSAs have been charged with responsibility for ensuring that staff employed by their independent contractors are adequately trained for their jobs. Some FHSAs have taken this responsibility more literally than others, and have worked pro-actively to stimulate the provision of training for practice-employed staff at all levels. Others have stood back from the provider role and tried to monitor training provided locally. Unfortunately, apart from one or two notable exceptions, neither approach has been wholly satisfactory.

At TCV we were keen to develop an effective model of FHSA involvement in training which built upon the lessons learnt in Gwent. At the same time, Mid Glamorgan FHSA was anxious to encourage the provision of locally accessible high quality training for receptionists. Although the population of Mid Glamorgan is one of the highest in Wales, most live in comparatively isolated communities often served by single-handed practices. This means that practice staff were often working in small surgeries. The FHSA wanted to develop a training programme which could reach staff in these isolated communities, as experience had shown that they were reluctant to travel out of their own areas. When the FHSA reviewed their training uptake, they discovered that only a very small proportion of practice staff had been formally trained. Very often training opportunities were being taken up by a small number of enthusiasts, while the majority remained indifferent. For example, 60% of those receptionists who had been in post for more than seven years, had not previously attended any training course.

On this basis TCV began to work with the FHSA to develop both a programme and a delivery process. The FHSA took on the role of commissioner: they stipulated the outcomes they wanted – a high quality training programme which would be accessible to most practices. TCV put together a three-day course, a 'Train the Trainers Programme', to train six practice managers to deliver a receptionists training programme. The six practice managers were hand-picked by the FHSA on the basis of their knowledge, experience and effective management. The programme concentrated on building the confidence of these six to enable them to acquire skills in presenting information to large groups, and in facilitating small group learning.

The three day workshop included presentation skills (with video feedback), role play and group work skills.

By the end of the three days, the practice managers were ready to begin the next phase. The FHSA provided administrative support and helped the practice managers to offer Practice Receptionist Training Programmes (PRPs) from within their own surgeries. This meant that courses could be provided in areas of greatest need (rather than being restricted to whichever further education colleges might express an interest). It also meant that costs could be kept to a minimum. This was an important consideration, particularly at the outset of the programme when the practice managers were teaching in teams. TCV provided ongoing support via regular team meetings with the six practice managers to discuss progress and problems. Within six months the six practice managers were reviewing their own progress, re-organising their teaching patterns, and chivvying the FHSA for more support. For example they requested extra audio-visual aids and, as a result of this, an overhead projector was provided for one Health Centre, situated in a notoriously difficult area in terms of training uptake.

The programme was evaluated and practice managers who had sent receptionists on the PRP courses taught by the team of practice managers were asked about their views of the effectiveness of the training. Overall, 79% reported a positive change in the work performance and behaviour of their receptionists after attending. Specific gains mentioned included:

- increased confidence;
- better ability to communicate;
- increased knowledge; for example, of FHSA forms and their purposes;
- smoother running of the practice;
- improved attitudes towards, and coping strategies with, patients;
- improved teamworking skills;
- increased knowledge of how other practices worked.

These findings indicated that 'bringing the programme to the people' was an effective means of increasing the uptake of training programmes. Interestingly, the evaluation study shows that as receptionists went on to higher levels – to PRP2 and PRP3 – there was a corresponding willingness to travel greater distances. So, by providing the initial course near to home and surgery, receptionists were encouraged to travel in order to obtain further qualifications. As we had found in the Gwent pilot project, the competence-based approach empowered participants and reduced their anxieties about learning.

The programme clearly benefited reception staff and therefore it is anticipated it will benefit patients in the long run. It was seen by employing practice managers to be a good vehicle for correcting bad, and reinforcing good, working methods.

The programme also benefited the six practice manager/teachers. This group increased in confidence and competence throughout the programme, and continued to grow and develop as they taught the course over the following two years. This model of collaboration was successful because it played to the strengths of all participating parties:

- The FHSA was the agency best placed to identify training needs, and the agency that set the standards that training programmes needed to work towards.
- The practice managers were ideally placed to create a learning opportunity for receptionists, removed from the pressures of their own workplaces; they could encourage good practice by drawing on their own expertise and by helping the pupil receptionists to share their ideas and experiences.
- TCV was able to provide the missing link – the management and teacher training which empowered the practice managers to use and develop that expertise.

Subsequent developments

Building on the work undertaken at TCV, the Valleys Health Group, working in partnership with South Glamorgan FHSA, Gwent Commission, UWCM and NHS Staff College Wales, has been using a development approach which combines the two approaches, academic and competence, into one coherent and comprehensive programme.

Our experience with the development of practice managers is that real change in practices needs practical support as well as the input of information or education. This mirrors the conclusions drawn from an evaluation of the TCV Practice Advisory Service (see Chapter 2).

The combination of academic and competence learning in this new approach seems to be the most appropriate and cost-effective way to provide relevant and effective development channels in a locally accessible fashion. Our new programme has been devised to provide a strong underpinning knowledge element, geared to the specific problems of management in the PHC context, and the course has been accredited by UWCM. The knowledge elements are paralleled by a programme of activity designed to help participants acquire the skills to perform to national standards of competence. It thus provides a stepwise channel in which participants can begin by acquiring recognition of their competence to manage to nationally recognised standards at an operational level (postgraduate certificate) and then move on to acquire strategic level competence (diploma level).

By structuring the development programme around national standards of performance, employer organisations have a ready-made measure of performance against which to structure their own reimbursement and reward strategies. This approach also helps to solve the present problem of how to develop meaningful pay structures in the face of the existing diversity of qualifications and responsibilities of the current practice management postholders. Individual employees now have a benchmark against which to build their own continuing professional development. The programme is beginning to pay dividends in the form of quantifiable improvements in management within the practices of participants.

Discussion

On the whole, FHSA staff had neither the resources, qualifications nor experience either to adequately provide comprehensive training programmes themselves, or to monitor and evaluate other training provided locally. For many FHSAs the training of those employed by practices has been a low priority.

However, even in areas where independent development projects have been able to contribute to educational programmes, progress in developing and establishing such programmes has been bedevilled by problems of competition and ownership. There has been an explosion of local programmes as colleges try to tap available new markets, all ostensibly providing management development opportunities. This has meant that individual practice managers are faced with a bewildering range of educational opportunities, but have had little in the way of methods by which to evaluate them. All this has hindered the establishment of a recognised and relevant development pathway for practice staff.

Most FHSAs have missed a golden opportunity to provide some sort of path through this maze. Contributing to the quality assurance process of local educational programmes would have been a good way for FHSAs to support aspiring practice staff. Arguably, providing clear guidance or advice about development opportunities available in a locality could be the best use of scarce development resources in the new Health Commissions.

The development of an appropriate career structure and an accredited career development pathway for practice managers and receptionist staff remains an urgent priority in PHC, as it does for other PHC practitioners. At the same time, policy changes and service development initiatives mean that there will always be a need for short courses aimed specifically at helping practices to implement proposed changes. If the full benefits of a PHC-based health service are to be realised, then considerable attention will need to be paid to the broader educational and development needs of practice managers and others working in the PHC setting.

The development work described in this chapter, combining the two key elements of knowledge and competence, provides some indication of the needs of practice managers and the ways in which these needs can be met through partnership activities between education providers, practice managers and HAs.

Reference

The Management Charter Initiative (1991) *Crediting Competence*. HMSO, London.

Chapter 4

Promoting Health and Safety

Peter Ganesh

Health and safety in the primary health care setting has been largely ignored by those who need to be protected. Likewise, many of those whose job it is to implement health and safety statutory regulations are themselves ignorant of the law. Many find it extremely confusing, which is not surprising given that health and safety legislation is some of the most complex on the statute books. Nevertheless there are handbooks available to guide the manager, Health and Safety Executive (1994) and Dewis (1995), for example.

This legislation covers many facets of everyday life in PHC including, for example, the use of computer screens, the handling and storage of substances such as bleach and correcting fluid, and the availability of first aid to workers.

Health and safety begins with the Health and Safety at Work Act, 1974. This is the umbrella under which the majority of health and safety legislation is enacted. The best place to start is Section 2(3) of this Act. This states that if you employ more than five persons, you must: 'prepare and bring to the employees' notice a written statement that sets out the organisation's policy on health and safety and the means to implement that policy.'

So, the question arises: to what extent are those responsible for PHC aware of this responsibility? At the spring meeting of the Royal College of General Practitioners in 1991, it was reported that a survey had revealed: 'that few GPs are aware of their statutory duties in regard to health and safety' (Williams, 1991). Locally, I had gained similar evidence from straw polls of practice managers, and from participants on the Mid Glamorgan Practice Receptionist Training Programme, of a lack of knowledge about health and safety.

The survey

This worrying evidence led me to approach TCV with a proposal for a more systematic study of this issue. This was accepted and I was appointed as a part-time management fellow with TCV. This study was conducted in Mid Glamorgan over a seven month period between February and August 1993.

A questionnaire was sent to all 106 practices in Mid Glamorgan (Ganesh, 1993). This was designed primarily to gauge the existing level of knowledge on health and safety matters. However, it was also intended to be a prompt to practices to look at their health and safety policies and procedures. The practices were given two weeks to complete and return the questionnaire prepaid to the TCV office in Cardiff. A total of 49 (46%) did so. Of these, 32 (65%) had over five employees.

Of the practices that returned the questionnaire, only half had a written health and safety policy. Few realised that, for those practices with five or more employees, there is a fine of up to £2,000 for failure to have one. Thus a number were in breach of the legislation.

In addition to responsibilities towards employed members of staff, the Act also places responsibilities on employers for staff who work from their premises but are not their employees. Section 4(2) of the Act states that: 'Controllers of premises have a duty to ensure as far as reasonably practicable that people who are not employees, but who use their premises as a place of work are not exposed to risks to health and safety.'

This means that, should health visitors or district nurses (or other members of the PHCT) work from, or in, a practice's premises, the practice has a duty towards them regarding their health and safety. To ensure this and to undertake other duties designated under the Act, a senior member of staff should be nominated as the Health and Safety Officer, someone who has delegated powers to enforce health and safety within the practice. If the practice manager is appointed as this officer, however, this does not mean that employers can forget their responsibilities, for Section 2 of the Act states: 'it shall be the duty of every employer to ensure so far as it is reasonably practicable the health, safety and welfare at work of all employees'.

In fact, only 16 practices (33%) had such a designated officer. Of these 16 officers, only one was an employer, a partner in the practice. Ten were practice managers and five were practice nurses or receptionists.

Although two in three practices knew that the Health and Safety Executive is responsible for enforcing health and safety legislation, ten thought this rested with the FHSA or the DHA.

Under the Control of Substances Hazardous to Health regulations (COSHH), employers must undertake a 'suitable and sufficient assessment' of the risks to health and safety created by exposure to any substance, and must prevent the exposure of employees to substances hazardous to their health. In PHC, people are exposed to a vast array of substances ranging from cleaning liquids to body fluids. The survey revealed that one in three practices had not heard of COSHH, nor did they know how to undertake an assessment of the workplace. Only 12 practices (24%) had undertaken an assessment within the past year. This is disappointing given the publicity given to COSHH by the Health and Safety Executive when the regulations were introduced in 1990. The local DHA had formed a Quality Team to monitor health and safety and was keen for this team to help GPs with COSHH.

Sharps and waste disposal are often given little thought and yet this is an area of health and safety that can present the most risk to both employees, patients and visitors to a surgery. There should be a written sharps policy in every practice, covering storage of container boxes, prevention of public access, marking, replacement and disposal arrangements. The survey revealed that 35 (71%) had a written policy, the majority taking part in the scheme run by the local FHSA. This is evidence of the potentially important role that the FHSA can play in ensuring health and safety standards in PHC.

The Electricity Regulations place a duty on employers to have safe electrical systems at the place of work and to check them regularly. Thirty of the responding practices (61%) were not aware of these regulations.

According to RIDDOR, the Reporting of Injuries, Disease and Dangerous Occurrences Regulations 1985, every organisation should have an accident reporting book. Usually this should be based on Form BI/510 as laid out by these regulations. Only half of the respondents to the survey had heard of the RIDDOR regulations. Only one in four knew that a form had to be completed if, as a result of an accident, an employee is absent from work for more than three days. Two in three had an accident book.

The Health and Safety (Information for Employees) Regulations require employers to display a poster 'Health and Safety Law – What you should know'. Only 16 (33%) of the practices had one on display. Two in three are in breach of the law by not having one.

The Workplace (Health, Safety and Welfare) Regulations require a sufficient number of thermometers to be provided to monitor the temperature of the workplace. A total of 20 (41%) of the practices had none. Only 37 respondents (76%) knew that the minimum temperature allowed in a workplace is 16 degrees centigrade.

Discussion

These findings indicate that most practices have some knowledge of health and safety, but that there is still a vast area of ignorance about the relevant regulations and legislation. Health and safety is not newsworthy unless it involves loss of life or limb, or unless a GP faces court action over a breach of the law.

Having analysed the findings of the questionnaire, there appear to be three main areas in which practices could be helped with health and safety management. First, many practices lack expertise in drawing up and implementing safety policies and procedures. The health and safety statement that these practices should have produced in compliance with the 1974 Act, should be a 'living' document, one that changes as the practice develops. Despite this, half of the respondents had not drawn up a policy. Second, more than half the practices had no plans to undertake an assessment in accordance with COSHH. Third, most practices did not understand the RIDDOR procedures.

Clearly training courses are needed. These could be organised by HAs using available resources or by buying in outside expertise. These courses need not be very time-consuming. Health and safety policies and procedures, together with RIDDOR, could be covered in one half day. The COSHH Regulations are more complex as they involve assessments of premises, and they may need one whole day. There are a great many substances in use in general practice and one suggestion is that a central database should be established in each area. While this is a good idea in the long term, it will take considerable time and effort to discover who uses what, and to identify the implications for employees. In the meantime, the matter of health and safety in PHC should be taken up under continuing medical education. Leaflets could be obtained from the Health and Safety Executive and distributed to each practice. A quarterly or half-yearly health and safety newsletter could be produced by the HA or by a practice manager's group. By taking such simple and sensible measures, we might hope that practices will become better informed (and less vulnerable to legal action) and, in particular, that the health of those who use PHC services or who work in surgeries and health centres will not be endangered by negligent management.

References

Dewis, M. (1995) *Tolley's Health and Safety at Work Handbook.* Tolley Publishing, Croydon.

Ganesh, P. (1993) *Health and safety management in general practice within Mid Glamorgan.* TCV Project Report. TCV, Welsh Office, Cardiff.

Health and Safety Executive (1994) *Essentials of Health and Safety at Work,* 3rd edn. Health and Safety Executive, London.

Williams, N.R. (1991) *General practitioner knowledge of and compliance with health and safety legislation.* Lecture. Royal College of General Practitioners, Spring Meeting, Newcastle.

Chapter 5

Managing Time, Workload and Health-related Behaviour: GPs

Chris Hoddell and Robert Jones

There have been a few studies that have looked at stress in GPs, and at whom GPs consult when they themselves fall ill. However, there have been none that we have discovered which have looked at health-related behaviour and that attempt to link this with workload. There has been an increasing emphasis placed on preventive medicine in recent years, particularly since the 1990 GP Contract. We wondered if those whose role it is to give advice were taking note of it themselves: if GPs were practising what they were expected to preach.

Other studies have reported that increasing workloads and stresses have resulted from the 1990 GP Contract (Hannay *et al.*, 1992; Sutherland & Cooper, 1992). A more recent study of GP burnout has confirmed these findings. It has also produced evidence that part-time GPs are less likely to suffer from burnout than their full-time colleagues (Kirwan & Armstrong, 1995). This suggests that good time management might be important and this confirms the relevance of a second hypothesis that we addressed when we undertook this study in 1992: that this pressure would be more readily borne by those GPs who have management skills, especially skills in time management. The third hypothesis we considered was that these GPs were also more likely to have positive health-related behaviour.

The survey

Our study was based on a postal questionnaire sent to all the GPs in the TCV area. We included a post-paid addressed envelope for the reply. The study assessed the GPs' attitude to healthy behaviour by asking questions about exercise, diet, smoking and drinking. We also tried to estimate the relative workload of the GPs with questions about list-size, number of partners, hours worked, on-call commitment, and the percentage of patients for whom deprivation payments were received. A brief time management questionnaire was also included.

We sent out a total of 381 questionnaires and 204 were returned completed – a 54% response. There was considerable variation in response between the various parts of the TCV area, the highest being 76% and the lowest 33%. We could think of no obvious explanation for this variation. We were pleased with the overall response rate and attributed this to two factors: first, the questionnaire was easy to answer and took no more than five minutes or so to complete, and, second, it was about a subject of interest to GPs: themselves.

With regard to healthy behaviour, we found that GPs do claim to be practising what they preach. They compare favourably with the general population in terms of smoking, drinking outside safe limits, obesity and taking regular exercise (Table 5.1).

Table 5.1   Health-related behaviour

	GPs %	General population* %
Smokes	13	32
Drinks more than safe limits	10	20
Is obese	31	46
Takes regular exercise	50	34

* Source: Heartbeat Wales (1990)

The proportion of GPs who smoke is markedly below that of the general population. If we take class into account, the proportion that smoke is lower than the proportion (15.7%) in social class I in the general population in Wales (Heartbeat Wales, 1990). Despite this evidence of healthier than average behaviour, 11% of the GPs thought themselves to be unhealthy.

The respondents reported that they work a mean of nearly ten hours on an average day. We defined high workload as those working ten or more hours a day and spending more than two nights a week on call. We compared those with such a workload with those reporting a lower workload. We found that those GPs with a higher workload were less likely to take regular exercise (53% v. 61%) and to be able to relax in their free time without worrying about work (57% v. 74%), and they were more likely to smoke (13% v. 9%). None, however, drank more than the recommended safe limit.

The formula determining the receipt of deprivation payments is intended to reflect pressures on GPs from patients with high health service needs. Over half (52%) of the respondents reported that they received no deprivation payments. In contrast, 21% receive deprivation payments for more than a quarter of their practice population. Those working in practices receiving higher deprivation payments had a higher divorce rate than other GPs (10% v. 6%), were more likely to eat an unhealthy diet (29% v. 19%), and to be overweight (38% v. 30%). Time management scores were similar in both groups.

We identified a category of 102 GPs who scored high on the time management scores – the good time managers – and another of 48 GPs who scored low – the poor time managers. We found that, compared with poor time managers, good time managers were more likely to consider themselves healthy (94% v. 77%), to take regular exercise (54% v. 46%), and to eat a healthy diet (82% v. 67%). They were less likely to be overweight (28% v. 44%).

However, unexpectedly, they were also more likely to smoke (18% v. 8%), and more likely to drink in excess of the recommended limit (12% v. 8%) – perhaps they had more time to indulge!

Discussion

We had expected that there would be a close relationship between high workload and poor health-related behaviour. We did not find this to be the case, except in the areas of exercise and the ability to relax when not working.

The GPs with the higher workload would be expected to have less time to take regular exercise, but it would appear that they try to look after their health in other ways: by eating a healthy diet, by avoiding obesity and smoking, and by keeping their drinking within sensible limits. This finding is modified by the figures for those GPs working in areas of high deprivation who were slightly more likely to eat an unhealthy diet and to be overweight. Perhaps the higher stress caused by working in an area of high deprivation contributed to this and to the fact that these GPs were more likely to be divorced.

It was encouraging that the GPs scored above the general population in all areas of health-related behaviour in which we were able to make comparisons: the profession seems to be trying to lead by example. One particularly surprising finding was that almost a third of the GPs reported that they were teetotal. This finding might be explained by the relatively high number of Muslim Asian GPs in the TCV area who would be teetotal by reason of religious conviction.

We found analysis of workload difficult, and tried various formulae for calculating it. However, we were unable to find any satisfactory way of weighting the various factors that make up a high workload. For example, should high list size be more heavily weighted than being frequently on-call? How much emphasis should be given to high levels of deprivation? Other studies of GPs' workload tend to be far more detailed than ours, and therefore were of little help to us. In the end we feel our solution of comparing those who worked more than 10 hours a day and did more than two nights a week on call (the high workload group) with those who worked less than 10 hours a day and less than two nights on call a week (the lower workload group) to be the best compromise.

The large majority (93%) of our sample provide their own out-of-hours cover, almost certainly due to the fact that there is no deputising service available in most of the TCV area. It would have been interesting to compare our GPs with those in a more affluent area with full access to a deputising service. We suspect that bigger differences in health-related behaviour might be demonstrated between these two groups.

In these days of ever-increasing workload and ever more frequent reports of stress and stress-related illnesses in GPs, the finding that we felt to be most important and to be of most practical value, was that of the positive relationship between time management and health-related behaviour. This is an area in which something could be done to help GPs.

Conclusion

As a group, the GPs in this survey report more positive health-related behaviour than the general population.

We did not find a simple relationship between workload and healthy behaviour, but there were indications that GPs with a high workload are less likely to exercise and to be able to relax when away from work. Independently of this, good time management appeared to be a positive factor for healthy behaviour.

This survey suggests that an in-depth study of a group of GPs with a high workload and who are also poor time managers would be of great value. We would predict that this group would have the worst health-related behaviour.

We would also recommend the establishment of a further project in which (i) GPs were offered training in time management, and (ii) their health-related behaviour was assessed before and after this training. This would test the hypothesis that health-related behaviour is improved by training in time management.

References

Hannay, D., Usherwood, T. & Platts, M. (1992) Workload of general practitioners before and after the new contract. *British Medical Journal*, **304**, 615–8.

HeartBeat Wales (1990) *Recent Trends in Lifestyles 1985–1990*. Technical Reports 24 and 25. Health Promotion Wales, Cardiff.

Kirwan, M. & Armstong, D. (1995) Investigation of burnout in a sample of British general practitioners. *British Journal of General Practice*, **45**, 259–60.

Sutherland, V.J. & Cooper, C.L. (1992) Job stress, satisfaction, and mental health of GPs before and after the new contract. *British Medical Journal*, **304**, 1545–8.

Chapter 6

Establishing Professional Support Groups

Bill Bytheway, Stephanie Williams and Rosamund Bryar

One objective that TCV set itself was to identify people involved in primary health care in the TCV area who were isolated from other members of their occupations, disciplines or professional groups. It was obvious from our involvement with some less isolated groups, such as GPs in group practices or team midwives, that mutual support between people in similar positions was important and valued. Such groups provide peer support and a forum for the sharing of ideas and experiences which can then be taken back to the members' individual practice. In a more formal sense they can provide the setting for educational events which can lead to the development of individual practices. Moreover, by maintaining our commitment to teamwork we could help these relatively isolated people become more fully appreciated within their local PHCT or more responsive, in the case of the Nurse Educators Group, to the needs of PHCTs.

There were three groups to whom we gave particular attention: practice managers, solo (or single-handed) general practitioners and nurse educators. Typically there is at most one practice manager in a PHCT. This person, as shown in Chapter 3, has distinctive responsibilities. A solo GP is a doctor in a unique position. Many patients prefer the continuity of care that the solo GP can offer but the pressures of work, and the difficulties of gaining the expertise to cope with the changing demands being placed on them, can put the solo GP in a particularly stressful position. This is exacerbated by the view that changes in policy are often imputed as heralding the end of the solo GP. PHC nurse educators relate to PHC not as members of teams but in the development and provision of educational and training opportunities. Unlike their opposite numbers in medicine, the CME tutors who operate from a clinical base in general practice, they are based in departments of nurse education, in FHSAs, trusts and other settings and do not have the same established support and communication systems available to CME tutors. In addition, they are somewhat over-shadowed in departments of nurse education by the continuing emphasis in nurse education on secondary care.

Practice managers

In 1992, 65% of the 155 practices in the TCV area had practice managers in post. Many of these practices are located in isolated and tight-knit communities. There had been a tendency for receptionists to be promoted from within these practices. Their lack of experience of the organisation of other practices and the limited management training opportunities available to them, had contributed to a tendency for them to continue to do things 'the way they've always been done'.

On a number of occasions in the first few months of TCV, however, we were told about the isolation felt by some local practice managers and of their interest in meeting together to share solutions to common problems. Unfortunately the pressure of work which followed the 1990 GP Contract had meant that none had had the time or energy to regularly meet other managers or to take on the task of setting up a local practice managers' group. Moreover, the emphasis in the Contract on competition meant that some GPs actively discouraged their managers from contacting their opposite numbers in other practices.

To meet this need we decided to work with a small group of key individuals to create a forum for practice managers, the majority of whom were in the Mid Glamorgan section of the TCV area. The longer-term aim was to enable the forum to become self-sustaining.

Setting up the Group

TCV facilitated and supported the formation of the Mid Glamorgan Practice Managers Group which first met in January 1991. Fifteen managers attended the first meeting in Caerphilly. TCV offered to facilitate and support the formation of the Group and it was agreed that there should be monthly meetings. The participants decided that it would be better to meet in different practices in the area rather than in one fixed venue, and that external speakers should be invited to address relevant topics. It was agreed that meetings would be in the early evening and that TCV would provide light refreshments to pre-cede the formal part of the meetings. This enticed busy managers to attend straight from work at the end of evening surgery.

The Mid Glamorgan FHSA responded positively to the Group's formation and the General Manager addressed one of the first meetings. His acceptance of the invitation was a key factor in giving the Group a high profile early in its life and in drawing the attention of doctors as well as practice managers to its establishment. More importantly it gave a message to GPs and practice staff that this group of staff was recognised and valued at the highest levels of local FHSA management.

It was agreed that a letter should go to all practice managers and any senior receptionists who were, in effect, acting as managers, inviting them to join the Group and informing them of subsequent meetings.

The project was evaluated at the end of the first year and the general response was very positive. Ten meetings had been held and attendance numbers varied from 7 to 33. Topics included indicative prescribing amounts, business planning, computers, pension schemes and health and safety. Despite the advantages of visiting different premises, the costs and difficulties of travel prevented many from attending some of the meetings. Travel was the most difficult problem that managers faced in attending the meetings.

Development

By December 1991, a core of about twelve to fifteen regular attenders had formed. These practice managers were especially keen to develop their skills. They volunteered for other educational activities and were willing to encourage other managers to join the Group. One wrote the following comments for *ReValley*, the TCV newsletter:

'The most important function of the Group is sharing problems and worries and realising that they are the same as everybody else's.... We've really all become friends – you have the confidence to share downfalls with others, without feeling that you are the only one who makes mistakes.'

By the middle of 1992 it was becoming clear that the core members were taking increasing responsibility for organising the Group. For example, it was decided to establish four sub-committees (each made up of two neighbouring practice managers) who would then host meetings in rotation in four surgeries that were convenient for these meetings. The role of TCV was reduced to circulating the membership with details of the forthcoming meeting. In addition, notes of the discussions that took place at the previous meeting were also circulated. This was valued because most of the eighteen members found it difficult to attend all meetings. Those who were interested in the proceedings but lacked transport were nevertheless keen to be kept informed.

This second series of monthly meetings continued through from May 1992 to June 1993. Attendance ranged from 7 to 42. The highest figure was for a meeting also attended by GPs and practice nurses about the revised health promotion banding arrangements. The success of this meeting was a clear indication of the importance of multi-disciplinary training on the implications for all practice staff of such major administrative changes.

Whenever a new development related to practice administration was mooted, whether it was a change in the way claim forms are laid out or a new emphasis on quality initiatives, FHSA representatives were invited to use the Group as a way of informing practices in some detail about the reasons for the proposed changes. In one instance, the preparation of Practice Development Plans, one meeting was insufficient and further seminars were sought from the FHSA.

The Group is now fully independent and self-supporting. It is an important two-way channel of communication between practice managers and the FHSA. For example, representatives from the Group sit on the Mid Glamorgan Local Planning Team which looks at training needs and standards for ancillary staff. This team meets monthly in order to commission training and to review the value for money of such courses. Similarly there is a representative of the Group on the Mid Glamorgan MAAG and, as a consequence, the Group has set up a subgroup looking specifically at audit issues. In 1995 the Group organised the highly successful first All Wales Practice Managers Conference attended by 148 practice managers from all corners of the Principality.

The Group remains vulnerable to the attempts of sectional interests to dominate, and to various vocational and professional organisations which are competing for the involvement of practice managers. But much of its strength derives from the fact that it is 'owned' by a wide range of participants who share a genuine commitment to the continuing professional development of the members. It may be that this commitment is best fostered by a group such as this, which is, and remains, independent.

Solo GPs

During the course of 1991, it was decided that TCV would appoint a number of short-term part-time clinical fellows (see Chapter 1). Shortly after making this decision, we were approached by Dr Edna Hayes, at that time working as a solo GP in Cardiff. She wanted help in completing the analysis of an all-Wales survey of solo GPs that she had recently undertaken.

There have been regular predictions that the solo GP is 'dying out'. The proportion in England and Wales fell from 43% in 1952 to 14% in 1980 (Fry, 1983). They have been popularly associated with poor practice, inadequate premises, poor out-of-hours cover, few teamwork skills in collaborating with other members of the PHCT and so on. Green (1993) has undertaken a study of the needs of single handed GPs in London. She recommended: clarification of the reimbursement priorities of FHSAs, more help in premises development, and a more positive approach from policy makers.

There was a high proportion of solo GPs in the TCV area: 12.2% compared with 8.3% in Wales as a whole. We wanted to establish contact with this important group of practitioners and saw the appointment of Dr Hayes as a clinical fellow as a valuable opportunity. She was appointed for twelve sessions with a remit to help organise and contribute to a meeting of solo GPs practising in the TCV area, and to produce a discussion paper to stimulate debate about the contribution and developmental needs of solo GPs.

Dr Hayes presented preliminary findings from her survey at the initial meeting held in August 1991. The discussion paper was issued the following February (Hayes, 1992). Her survey revealed that solo GPs in Wales as a whole were predominantly male and over 35 years of age. Their list sizes were variable. One in eight had fewer than 1,200 patients – the figure fixed for the Basic Practice Payment. Conversely, over half had list sizes of over 2,000, well above the figure of 1,700 which is considered ideal.

They all reported workload increases since the 1990 GP Contract, in all areas of practice except that of paid work outside the practice. Although help is available from other doctors, locums, assistants and the deputising service, only one in seven availed themselves of such relief. None had trainees. Seven out of eight received income through the postgraduate education scheme, just under half had joined the cost rent scheme for premises, and one in three received deprivation payments.

Most had reached at least the low targets for immunisation and cytology, and the majority offered a range of other services which they provided themselves: antenatal visits, over-75 health checks, minor surgery, and so on.

Their attitudes to the 1990 Contract were mixed. One in four thought that services for patients would improve, but only 9% felt that there would be any improvement in job satisfaction. Over half felt that solo GPs would disappear as a result of the Contract. One in five were pessimistic about their own future and over half were trying to share their practice with another doctor. One in four were anticipating a reduced income.

Setting up the Group

Eight doctors were able to attend the meeting arranged by Dr. Hayes in August 1991. Another sixteen had expressed interest but were unable to be present. A lively discussion followed her presentation, and it was decided that a series of further meetings should be arranged. These would include an educational element, thereby qualifying those who attended for their postgraduate education allowance. Dr Srivastava of Troedyrhiw agreed to chair these meetings and to liaise with TCV and the CME tutor. The representative of a pharmaceutical company agreed to sponsor the Group, support which was very much appreciated and contributed greatly to the enjoyment of the meetings.

Between November 1991 and June 1992, there were five further meetings. At the second, the participants were asked to identify issues that they felt should be examined in more detail. They listed five: patient education, teamwork in PHC, changes in community care policies, the anticipated increase in HIV-AIDS cases, and 'reaching the unreachables': people who do not attend clinics.

These topics were covered in subsequent meetings, and we endeavoured to vary the pattern in order to test out different strategies for attracting participation. Participants were asked to undertake preparatory work prior to each meeting. This included an audit exercise, identifying actions to improve patient education, and interviewing other members of the PHC team. We consider this to have been a crucial part of the educational programme, since practitioners were required to undertake activities within their practices which promoted teamwork, and which obliged them to relate what they learnt in the Group to the organisation of their practice. The suggestion that a member of the Group should lead a discussion led to three members taking up this challenge. All three drew upon practice-based experience before raising broader ethical or organisational issues.

Much use was made of anonymised case material or anecdotal evidence. On occasions the usefulness or relevance of this was challenged and then the discussion turned to matters of audit and how GPs might organise their knowledge, gained through experience, in order to promote and develop organisational change. The fifth meeting included outside speakers from the FHSA and the Social Services. Although a stimulating discussion followed, it seemed more divorced than the previous meetings from matters to do with practice.

At the end of the first year, there were 31 solo GPs on the mailing list, all but a few practising in Mid Glamorgan. Of these, seven had attended more than three of the meetings and another eight had attended one or two.

Development

Initially it had been decided that it would be inappropriate to open up the Group to other people who might be interested, since it was important that the solo GPs who took part felt they were in control of their group. Three were regularly accompanied by their wives or practice managers. They, together with one or two members of TCV and the pharmaceutical representative, constituted the only participants who were not solo GPs. After the first year, however, it seemed that a core had been established and that the Group had a clear sense of its purpose, both in regard to education and to mutual support. Having reached this situation, there was a discussion about the future of the Group.

TCV had been represented at every meeting, primarily fulfilling a facilitating role. In addition to this, TCV had undertaken the bulk of the administrative work that was involved. We felt that we could no longer sustain this commitment to what had become a well-established but comparatively small group. We indicated that TCV could only remain actively involved if there was some further development which might engage other practices or contribute significantly to the promotion of teamwork.

The Group was reluctant to lose the support of TCV and so it decided to invite GPs in two-partner practices to become members, and to issue invitations as appropriate to practice nurses, practice managers and other members of the PHCT.

Ten meetings followed between September 1992 and July 1993. These were well attended. Seven involved outside speakers, four from the FHSA. Practice nurses were invited to three of these meetings and practice managers to another one.

Solo GPs were not overwhelmed by GPs from two-partner practices. There were 37 GPs who attended at least one of the first five meetings. Of these 14 were solo, 17 came from two-partner practices and, interestingly, six came from three or four partner practices. To some extent this reflected the fact that GPs move between practices and that practices change in size. We should not imagine that all solo GPs are solo through choice or for the whole of their careers in practice.

The contrast between the two years is revealing. In the first, a close camaraderie was established within a small group of doctors who were comparatively isolated. It was clearly apparent that, through participation in the Group, they had gained confidence and benefited from mutual support. Nevertheless, they were reluctant to agree to the withdrawal of TCV. In the second year, they remained active participants, but the Group developed the ambiance of more traditional educational meetings, well attended and addressed by expert speakers. It is easy to conclude that the Group had become 'dependent' upon the support that TCV gave. What is probably nearer the truth though is that all of them were reluctant to assume an unfamiliar lead role which might place substantial demands upon their time.

The final meeting (before the withdrawal of TCV) was addressed by Dr Jameson, Vice-Chair of the UK-wide Small Practices Association and, with his encouragement, a decision was taken to establish a branch of this association in the South Wales Valleys. So, after two years of development work by TCV and the initial core of solo GPs, these practices were well placed to continue to raise the quality of their practice and to find ways of securing their place in the future provision of PHC in South Wales.

Nurse educators

The Nurse Educators Group was different from the two other Groups as it was established to meet the needs of a group of people who, in the main, were not working in PHC, but were nevertheless making an important contribution to nursing in PHC. Nursing (and midwifery) have played an important part in the development of PHC although this contribution may not have been fully recognised or utilised (NHSME, 1993; Bryar, 1994). Nursing and nurse education is still dominated by the secondary sector and PHC nursing still does not command the central place it should hold amongst nurses. An additional hindrance to the full contribution of nursing is the divisions between the many types of nurses working in PHC. These divisions militate against a coherent voice for the place of nursing in PHC development. Nurse educators providing education for nurses in PHC thus face a number of problems both from their educational colleagues and from the variety of needs presented to them by nurses in PHC settings.

The links between educational providers and their potential student populations are commonly weak and poorly developed. Courses and other events may not be responding to current and future educational needs of those in PHC. This problem was exacerbated in the TCV area by the number of educational providers serving sections of the five health authorities included in the area. This resulted in major difficulties in disseminating information about courses and other educational events to potential students. Lack of communication between educational providers also meant that there was potential for overlap or gaps in course provision. In addition nurse educators involved in PHC education are in a minority in departments of nurse education and may lack support and feel isolated amongst the large number of their colleagues whose work is focused on secondary care.

One of the aims of TCV was to investigate and respond to the educational needs of the PHC practitioners in the area. This aim was addressed in a number of ways, some of which are described in Chapters 3, 11 and 12. Through contact with the practitioners in the area TCV was in a position to identify their educational needs. It was appropriate that TCV met some of these needs directly through the provision of:

- study days, for example on immunisation;
- distance learning and supported learning, for example the course Community and Public Health in the Valleys;
- through other educational activities such as the TCV Conference.

However, it was impossible and also inappropriate for TCV to try to meet the needs of all the PHC professionals in the area. Rather TCV had a function in helping to make known to other providers the needs of practitioners in the area.

Setting up the Group

It was apparent that practitioners in the area lacked information about courses available to them, and that those involved in the provision of education for nurses in PHC had no forum where they could meet to share common interests. Therefore, in the second year of operation of TCV, a Group was established for all those involved in nurse education in the area. This included:

- lecturers from departments of nursing and midwifery in universities, the Polytechnic of Wales (now the University of Glamorgan), colleges of nursing and midwifery, and colleges of further and higher education;
- practice nurse facilitators from FHSAs;
- nurses in practice in the area who had responsibilities for continuing education;
- members of staff of TCV.

The majority of members were drawn from the departments of nursing and midwifery, also from FHSAs, and four members were practitioners with responsibilities in relation to meeting the continuing education needs of nurses in their area of practice (a model similar to that of the CME tutor but one which is poorly developed in nursing).
The objectives of the Group were:

- to provide a forum for nurse educators in the TCV area to meet and exchange ideas;
- to provide a route for the identification of educational needs of nurses in the area and for the dissemination of information about the educational needs of nurses identified by TCV;
- to provide a forum for the development of joint educational initiatives;
- to provide a forum for the dissemination of information from TCV research projects which might be of relevance to nurse educators.

Development

The Group met on six occasions over a period of 22 months, with a membership of 32 people some of whom attended each meeting. Between 7 and 13 members attended the meetings which were held at the TCV offices. Agendas included the regular exchange of information about new courses, areas of development work and needs identified in the area. In addition, a presentation was made at each meeting on one of the TCV projects which had particular relevance for the Group. Many of the members of the Group had been involved at various stages of the project on the educational needs of practice nurses (see Chapter 11) and this session generated a great deal of discussion. A presentation on the standards of care project (see Chapter 8) led to the identification of a gap in the provision of information on this topic in local courses and invitations to Jennie Gill to contribute to a number of courses in the area. These presentations also had an educational purpose for the clinical fellows who had the opportunity of describing their findings to a supportive group prior to presentations to less familiar groups.

Benefits of the Group meetings were considered to be the opportunity to meet others involved in nurse education from other institutions and organisations whom they would not normally meet; reduction of isolation; making contacts with others and sharing information about what was going on in the area. Interestingly, greater awareness of multidisciplinary approaches was generated for those attending this uni-disciplinary group. It was considered that the Group had contributed to the identification of educational needs, in particular the needs of practice nurses, and had in some cases reinforced information that was already available about the needs of certain groups. The Group did not develop any joint educational initiatives but there was considerable sharing of information about developments in different places including the timing and provision of places for staff from different areas on courses. The development of educational initiatives takes a considerable amount of time and may have been something that could have been achieved by the Group in the long term. The Group was seen as particularly helpful in bringing together people who were outside educational institutions but who had responsibilities for education with people who were in centres of education. There was some disappointment amongst members about the lack of attendance at the meetings of key PHC nurse educators.

The Group was administered by TCV and all meetings were held at the TCV offices in Cardiff, a location which was accessible to all members. Group meetings were infrequent and, although a core group of people attended and a number of these were prepared to continue the meetings following the ending of TCV, support for the Group was not robust enough for the meetings to continue. Changes in the educational climate between 1990 and 1991 with the increase in competition between educational providers might also have contributed to the lack of organisational support for staff to attend such meetings. The ending of TCV also removed the area focus and concern with the educational needs of nurses beyond the boundaries of individual organisations.

Conclusion

The support of individuals in uni-disciplinary groups may initially appear to run counter to the aim of developing teamwork amongst members of the different occupational groups working in PHC. Our experience demonstrates that rather the opposite may be the outcome. The practice manager, general practitioner or nurse educator isolated from members of their own peer group may lose sight of their own particular skills and unique contribution, may maintain traditional activities which others in the peer group have discarded, and may feel devalued in the wider PHCT. Membership of a unidisciplinary group provides the opportunity for the sharing of common concerns, the exploration of new approaches and support from people who share a common occupational background. With this support, and new knowledge, members of the Groups were able to develop their own practice and contribute to the enhancement of the work of their own and other PHCTs. Teamwork was also developed through activities held at the group meetings as discussed above.

TCV provided the impetus for the establishment of the three Groups and considerable attention was paid to the process of maintenance of the Groups following the ending of TCV. Two of the Groups continued while the third did not. From this experience it can be suggested that groups are more likely to continue where the members have clear benefits from attending, where the group has external support and where transfer of responsibility has been carefully planned. In the case of the Practice Managers Group, members obtained support from the Group but were also involved in the ongoing development of educational courses, the Group had support from the local FHSA and responsibility for the organisation was shared between a sub-group of the members. In the case of the GPs, enlargement of group membership and alignment with a national organisation combined with the educational and social benefits of the group ensured its survival. The Nurse Educators Group provided those attending with benefits but it had no outside support and may have had some institutional opposition to its continuation. Geographical distance between members may also have inhibited continuation as might the absence of key nurse educators from the area at meetings. The membership of this group crossed many organisational and geographical boundaries and it is perhaps only possible for a body such as TCV which transcends such boundaries to facilitate the meetings of such a group.

References

Bryar, R. (1994) *Nursing Outcomes of Teamcare Valleys.* Welsh Office, Cardiff.
Fry, J. (1983) *Present State and Future Needs in General Practice.* MTP Press, Lancaster.

Green, J. (1993) *The problems faced by single-handed general practitioners.* Report for the South East Thames Primary Care Development Fund. Department of General Practice, UMDS, London.

Hayes, E. (1992) *Single-handed General Practitioners and the new Contract.* TCV Discussion Paper No. 9. TCV, Welsh Office, Cardiff.

NHSME (1993) *New World, New Opportunities. Nursing in Primary Health Care.* DoH, London.

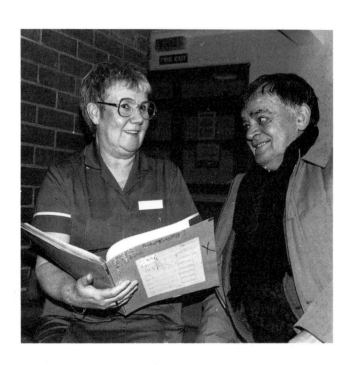

Section 2

Audit

In its early days, in 1990 and 1991, TCV was heavily involved in the production and provision of an all-Wales course on audit for GPs and practice managers. Audit activities became an important element of the TCV programme. Ajay Thapar, for example, developed the idea for his project (reported in Chapter 16) while participating in the all-Wales course, and then auditing the care his practice provided for asthma patients.

The four chapters in this section provide examples of how TCV became involved in developing and supporting audit projects. Whether these centre on clinics or professional practice, the aim was to establish in practice the cycle of observation, standard setting, agreeing criteria, gathering data, making comparisons with standards and implementing change.

The needs of patients with some chronic conditions are increasingly being met through PHC clinics. Chapter 7 describes an initiative intended to improve and develop diabetic care in general practice through the utilisation of national standards in the establishment of clinics. By auditing current practice, and then encouraging practices to introduce diabetic clinics, the project demonstrated that, with support, PHC can take on responsibilities that have previously rested with hospital-based clinics. This project also illustrates the vital role of the practice nurse in PHC and the importance of ongoing education in the development of standards of patient care.

Raising the quality of PHC services is an important element in the general development of PHC. One way of achieving this is through the PHCT setting its own standards and implementing procedures for monitoring progress. Chapter 8 presents a case study of such an initiative: the development of a 'Well Elderly' clinic. It offers lessons in how teams can be assisted in raising standards - and how raising standards promotes teamwork.

Each profession has its own particular skills and, in the development of management procedures, these need to be properly measured. The practice of health visiting is notoriously difficult to measure. How can a measurement tool be developed in relation to the content and quality, rather than the quantity, of health visiting? Chapter 9 considers the question of whether and how inter-personal skills (IPSs) in health visiting can be measured. It shows how health visitors and their clients share certain common values with regard to health and differ in other respects. This project addresses the important issue of health promotion and quality of practice. Traditionally much audit data collected in PHC has been concerned with indices which are counted. Relationships are central to the practice of all PHC practitioners and measurement of effective care also needs to include measurement of the qualitative aspects of care, whether that care is provided by GPs, receptionists or health visitors.

The last chapter in this section demonstrates the contribution to audit of information gathered by observing practice. Repeat prescribing has traditionally received little attention and is an area of continuing poor practice concerned both with clinical care and management systems within a practice. How can MAAGs and FHSAs help doctors to improve their effectiveness? Is there a conflict between the realities of practice and current policy concerns regarding the regulation and control of prescribed medication? How should the doctor respond to patient expectations? Chapter 10 touches on these questions in reporting on how a project undertaken by a practising GP moved from an interest in continuing medication to the organisation of repeat prescribing systems. Again it was through audit exercises that GPs came to realise the need for change. This chapter also provides an insight into the experience of TCV for one Valleys GP.

The chapters in this section are all concerned with the practicalities of raising standards of care in PHC. All the projects were undertaken by PHC practitioners demonstrating that, given support and time to develop audit systems, practitioners can devise and develop a wide range of approaches to audit in practice.

Chapter 7

Auditing GP Diabetic Clinics

Diane Wallis

The original idea for a project on GP diabetic clinics came from the consultant diabetologist based in East Glamorgan General Hospital. She was interested in developing general practice diabetic care having recognised that, subject to there being good communication and liaison between the hospital service and those providing care in the community, this held many advantages for all concerned. Prior to the introduction of the 1990 GP Contract, she had been working to these ends with a few local GPs for some years. Of a total of 31 practices in Rhondda and Taff Ely, the areas of Mid Glamorgan which jointly form the catchment area for the hospital, there were four practices running diabetic clinics in 1990. These four had been set up in conjunction with the consultant diabetologist and they used a protocol which they had jointly developed for shared-care.

The, then newly introduced, 1990 GP Contract led to remuneration for GPs on a sessional basis for providing diabetic care, amongst other things, in general practice. This led to a huge growth in the number of practices deciding to provide diabetic care throughout the country, and South Wales was no exception. By the summer of 1993 there were 25 practices in Rhondda and Taff Ely running GP diabetic clinics.

As the growth in GP diabetic care took place, it was recognised that there was a fall in numbers attending the hospital diabetic clinic. Although this was to be expected in an environment where general practice diabetic care was being provided, there was some anxiety on the part of the hospital personnel as no communication was developing between the hospital and the new clinics, and nothing was known of the standard of care being provided.

Launching the TCV project

The TCV project began against this background: a time of great change in general practice, and insufficient communication between the providers of diabetic care in the hospital and the community. The project started in the spring of 1991 and ran until TCV closed in the late summer of 1993. The initial objectives were:

- to visit all the practices in Rhondda and Taff Ely in order to discover their present activities and future plans regarding the provision of diabetic care;
- to encourage the use of a standard protocol for general practice diabetic care;
- to provide hands-on assistance for practices wishing to start diabetic clinics or to further develop the care they were providing;
- to encourage the audit of diabetic care in general practice.

The first visits were to the six practices in the Rhondda Valleys which had set up their own clinics following, or in anticipation of, the introduction of the new funding arrangements. Information gained from these visits was used to assess the type of input which was likely to be required in other practices. The main findings from these first visits were:

- the main concerns of personnel running these clinics were organisational: too much paperwork, busy clinics, ineffective record keeping;
- there had been little attempt at planning the approach to providing diabetic care in general practice;
- there was a lack of awareness of services available for diabetics, for example from dieticians and chiropodists;
- none of the clinics had properly organised annual review examinations;
- none had a functioning diabetic register;
- there was minimal use of HbAlc tests, tests that are required to monitor diabetic control;
- all felt that they were providing good clinical care.

These findings were used as the basis for subsequent visits and for the development of resources for the practices. All 31 practices in the Rhondda and Taff Ely areas were visited during the course of the project, and the input varied according to need, receptiveness, and current level of diabetic care provided. After each initial visit a short report was prepared and sent to the practice, outlining the issues which had been identified and the support which had been offered. Ongoing input from TCV was then arranged as necessary. Clinics continued to spring up during the course of the project and not all of the practices chose to avail themselves of the support being offered. Every practice had to be approached with tact and on its own terms. Some refused all offers of help whereas others asked for and received the maximum amount available.

At the same time, approaches were made to the other relevant health professionals concerned with diabetic care and to the appropriate managers. In particular, the referral criteria to dietitians, chiropodists, diabetic liaison sisters, the hospital diabetic clinic, ophthalmologists and renal physicians, were clarified and this information passed back to practices. Two diabetic liaison sisters were in post and working closely with the hospital diabetic teams. They were keen to be involved in the development of general practice diabetic care and one became a short-term clinical fellow with TCV, undertaking a project involving the education of practice nurses about diabetic care (Davies, 1993). Links were developed with the hospital biochemistry laboratory to prepare them for an increase in HbAlc samples and to lobby for their support for a specimen pick-up service for the practices in the District. Attempts were made to gain the support of the LMC, FHSA, MAAG and DHA. All except the FHSA were generally supportive of the project.

Providing support

The importance of good organisation in general practice diabetic care cannot be over-emphasised. If it is not there then whatever care is provided will be sub-standard. For many of these practices, providing a pro-active service for patients was a new experience. Most of the clinics in the Rhondda and Taff Ely were run by practice nurses, with various degrees of input from GPs. The best practices had good lines of communication and clear ideas of the tasks which they had to perform in order for the clinic to run smoothly. I actively encouraged this sort of team approach. In some, difficult internal practice relationships meant there was a lack of co-ordination between the GP, practice nurse and administrative staff.

A variety of problems were encountered by practices without an organised approach to their diabetic care:

- practices without a diabetic register were unable to provide planned diabetic care;
- clinics with no call and re-call system, based on a register, saw the same patients over and over again, but were not able to review the total diabetic population in the practice;
- some patients continued to attend the hospital while also attending the practice clinic. This doubled the number of times the patient was seen with little or no advantage to the patient.

Audits

Following the initial fact-finding and offers of support, practices were encouraged to perform audits of their diabetic care. All practices were approached again and visited in order to discuss a potential audit. There were two types of audit suggested: baseline audits prior to starting a diabetic clinic, and audits of clinics which were already in progress. No practice had spontaneously performed an audit before starting a diabetic clinic. Wherever possible, the practice staff were encouraged to collect the data themselves and I would then analyse this for them and produce a report. In many practices, however, I undertook some or all of the data collection. On no occasion was a GP involved in collecting data. It was the practice nurse who undertook this task in the practices which managed to collect their own clinic data. Many of the practice nurses were not given extra time by their employing GPs in order to perform the audits. This was despite the fact that the local MAAG was willing and able to provide funds for the practice nurse to be employed for extra sessions. Only one practice took up this opportunity.

Baseline audits were used to enable the practice to see what improvements were necessary. Common findings were that only about two in three diabetic patients were attending the hospital for diabetic care, and that only small numbers of appropriate tests were performed by the practice on the known diabetic population.

In two practices it was possible to perform an audit before the clinic started and again after its first year. These showed great improvements in the care that was offered. The ascertainment rate also rose dramatically as practice staff became aware of more people with diabetes.

Audits were planned in fourteen established clinics and seven of these were completed. These were used to reveal strengths and weaknesses and to encourage staff to further develop the services they offered.

Development

Several reports on the activities of this project were produced and circulated to GP practices and other relevant bodies (Wallis, 1991). Resources for practices were also developed:

- a fact sheet on the use of HbAlc tests, produced in conjunction with the biochemistry staff;
- a practical guide to starting and running a GP diabetic clinic (Wallis, 1993a);
- a practical guide to auditing diabetic care in general practice (Wallis, 1993b).

It seems likely that the types of problems uncovered by this project exist in other districts, especially where there is a relatively deprived population. It is also likely that others who intend to embark on a 'diabetes in general practice' development project would have similar experiences.

At the close of the project, the funding arrangements were again about to change, and many of the practices were voicing the opinion that it would not be cost-effective for them to continue providing diabetic care for their patients. Others, however, have gained a lot from running these clinics and had every intention of continuing with them.

General practice or hospital care for people with diabetes?

The treatment of people with diabetes is ideally suited to general practice in the majority of cases, especially for those with straightforward maturity onset diabetes. The reason is that it is common, fairly easy to treat, and the annual examination required to check the condition of a patient is easy to perform.

Many GPs do not treat their diabetic patients in general practice. There are several reasons for this. Hospital physicians have traditionally regarded the treatment of diabetes as their domain and are often unwilling to discharge patients to the care of their GP. Because of this, many GPs have become de-skilled and wary of treating diabetes because they are told that it is too difficult. It does take some extra effort to treat diabetics in general practice, but most of the care and checks are simple and straightforward. The main stumbling block appears to be the eye examination required for detecting diabetic retinopathy. This does require some practice and skill on the part of the GP. More generally, as is argued in Chapter 12, the management of eye problems in PHC causes some difficulty and there is a clear need for training opportunities to be developed in this area.

The lessons learned

On the whole, this project fulfilled its objectives in that all practices in the two target areas were visited and offered support. They were encouraged to adopt a standardised approach, and many performed audits of their diabetic care (Greenhalgh, 1994). In retrospect there are several lessons which have been learned from this project. I hope they will help others embarking on similar projects. I have certainly learned a lot about development work in general practice which I will use in my career in public health medicine.

- The project developed as it progressed rather than was planned at its inception. It was not possible to predict the degree of input and education which was required. The types of supporting documents which were needed could only be determined after considerable practical work had been done. This has implications for project commissioning and management.

- There are so many issues involved in developing diabetic care that a multi-disciplinary team would have been better placed to provide the development support. Although attempts were made to work in conjunction with the local diabetic liaison sisters, PHC facilitators and the MAAG, there was a varying degree of commitment and expertise available from these sources. As a result, the project was largely run by myself, a general practice-trained doctor with extra training in diabetic care.
- TCV had many problems in establishing itself as a credible force. It would be more effective to base the sort of project described in this chapter in an HA, rather than in a quasi-independent university project. The complete lack of support from the local FHSA for this project was extremely damaging.
- In the limited time available, it would have been easier to concentrate on just one issue, such as developing registers, assessing educational needs or undertaking audit. There were so many aspects of work which needed developing that it was very easy to fall into the trap of trying to be all things to all people.
- It took at least two years to identify the practical advice and assistance that was needed to set up and audit diabetic clinics in general practice.
- Because of the short-term nature of the project, it is impossible to evaluate it in terms of improvements for diabetic patients. The audits showed that the change between the care prior to setting up a clinic and that achieved after one year of clinical operation was enormous, but this could only be measured in terms of process and structure, not in terms of outcome.
- It is difficult to make people change their practice. In particular, it was difficult to balance a helpful and supportive attitude to the practices against the fact that on many occasions the care they were providing was poor. As a member of an outside organisation with no statutory responsibility or control over practice funding there was little that I could do in terms of sanctions or inducements. The audits, however, were very helpful in achieving some change.
- Hospital diabetologists and GPs do not have the same perception of priorities in diabetic care provision. It is very important to get the support and the views of both sides in a project like this. One of the strengths of this project was that I was accepted by both hospital and practice teams.
- Practising PHC professionals have a heavy and varied workload. This must not be forgotten when planning this type of project which looks at only one specific area of care. Project workers need to understand the demands placed on the time of PHC professionals.
- Educational support is very important if real changes are to be made in general practice diabetic care. GPs and practice nurses need

training in the care of diabetic patients. The wider PHCT may also need developing if care is to be really effective.

In summary, this project has demonstrated that, with initial support, and in liaison with a diabetologist, GP practices are able to take on primary responsibility for the routine care of diabetic patients.

References

Davies, K. (1993) *Review of the training needs of practice nurses in diabetes health care in Rhondda Health Unit*. TCV Project Report. TCV, Welsh Office, Cardiff.

Greenhalgh, P.M. (1994) *Shared Care for Diabetes. A Systematic Review*. Occasional Paper 67. Royal College of General Practitioners, London.

Wallis, D. (1991) *General practice diabetic care in the Rhondda Valleys – a report on stage one of the TCV diabetic mini-clinic project*. TCV Project Report. TCV, Welsh Office, Cardiff.

Wallis, D. (1993a) *A practical guide to starting and running a general practice diabetic clinic*. TCV Guidelines. TCV, Welsh Office, Cardiff.

Wallis, D. (1993b) *Auditing diabetic care in general practice*. TCV Guidelines. TCV, Welsh Office, Cardiff.

Chapter 8

Setting Standards and Developing Quality

Jennie Gill

Quality and standard setting has been a central issue in the development of health care since the mid-1980s. In 1989 the establishment of a service-wide framework for medical audit, to be in place in general practice by April 1992, was a major priority in the White Paper *Working for Patients* (DoH, 1989). The Welsh Office document *A Quality Health Service for Wales* proposed an extension of this commitment to all members of the PHCT:

> 'While initially the focus may be on medical audit, primarily involving the medical profession, development is often dependent on a multidisciplinary approach or clinical audit.' (Welsh Office, 1990:25)

> 'Clinical audit, involving all members of the primary health care (PHC) team, should be a natural extension of medical audit.' (Welsh Office, 1990:16)

Clinical audit may be carried out in a number of different ways, one of which starts with the establishment of multidisciplinary standards of care. I already had an interest in audit when I joined TCV as a full-time clinical fellow and, as my interest was mirrored by that of practices in the area, I was able to undertake a project on audit while at TCV. The project was carried out between January 1991 and November 1992. The following outlines why the project was undertaken, the methods used, some solutions to the problems encountered, conclusions and some recommendations.

Monitoring standards of care

In my practice as a health visitor, over the three years prior to my appointment with TCV, I had used standard setting as an effective method of solving health visiting problems. However, I found that there were limitations to this unidisciplinary approach and I came to appreciate the need for an alternative which involved a multi-disciplinary group of professionals setting standards for activities in which they were collectively involved.

I also found that teamwork is not the most striking feature of PHCTs. Often the word is used solely to aid stratification, like 'flock' to describe a group of birds or 'herd' to describe a group of elephants. 'Team' usually describes a collection of people who look after a specific group of patients, generally those who are registered with a particular GP. It does not necessarily imply that they collaborate, communicate or value each other.

It appeared likely that, within the PHCT, planning and evaluating care for the practice population could not only improve the quality of patient care, but it might also provide the opportunity for improved teamworking and collaboration. As a King's Fund report comments:

> 'Establishing effective communication between all parties is a sound basis for constructing collaborative systems that work successfully. For high quality community care to become a reality mutual understanding and practical response are both essential.' (King's Fund Centre, 1990:68)

Having decided that multidisciplinary standard setting was worthy of examination, I had to choose a suitable method of investigation. This method should enable me to achieve my objective – to improve both the quality of patient care and teamworking. As far as general practice is concerned, the Royal College of General Practitioners contrasted standard setting activities in Britain which started at the level of individual doctors and practice, with that of the USA where legislation has resulted in imposed external standards (RCGP, 1985:3).

The American experience has shown that imposed standards will tend to be resisted by doctors but that, despite this, minimal standards are extended to many more doctors because legislation requires it. The British method of self-regulation may be criticised as being limited by the lack of career or financial incentives to perform well. On the plus side, however, self-regulation is more likely to secure compliance because the standards are agreed by the doctors themselves. Nurses have also developed methods of critically examining their work. Several preformulated tools have been designed to monitor nursing care (for example, Monitor, Qualpacs, Slater, see Parsley & Corrigan, 1994) but, when assessed in this way, nurses have no involvement in setting the standards and often resent this somewhat autocratic approach.

Morison has argued that it can generate: 'resentment, lack of initiative and unwillingness to accept that problems exist' (1992: 715).

Nurses, like doctors, prefer to be involved in developing their own measuring tools. The RCN Dynamic Standard Setting System (DySSSy) has provided the framework for nurses to set their own standards and criteria (RCN, 1990). Because it is underpinned by a philosophy of ownership and involvement in the decision making, it is the preferred method of audit for many nurses.

The DySSSy approach involves small groups of nurses working together to set standards relevant to their practice. The format used is the Donabedian model of structure, process and outcome (Donabedian, 1966). The extent to which the desired outcome is achieved is measured in terms of observed care delivery, practitioner's judgement and the patient's perception of the quality of care received. As the DySSSy method is also simple and flexible and was the most popular within nursing at the time of this study, I decided to use the basic framework and adapt it where necessary.

The project: standard setting for a 'Well Elderly' clinic

One of the practices which I visited as part of the initial visits to practitioners in the area, presented me with an ideal venue for carrying out the project and a relevant topic to audit. Staff identified falling standards of care in their 'Well Elderly' clinic, and they felt that this activity might benefit from a multidisciplinary, problem-solving approach in which team members would set a standard which they could all agree, and which was at a level they all wished to attain. As peer assessment would be used for evaluation it was vital that all members were confident enough to express their views. It was agreed that my role was to create a climate in which, by working together, team members would develop trust in their colleagues' judgement of what was an acceptable standard of working practice and care.

At the beginning of the project, several meetings were held with various members of the core planning group for the clinic. From a large number of people deemed to have an interest in the clinic, a small group was chosen to set the standard, with the remainder to be called on when necessary for advice, information and education. Our standard-setting group comprised the community sister, a GP, a health visitor and a receptionist. I was included as facilitator.

From the start, it was difficult to arrange meetings when everyone was available. Often the only way to move forward was for the few present to discuss a subject at length, make suggestions, and then put these to other members of the core team. The one time when all staff were together was during the clinic and decisions were often taken on these occasions. Sometimes it only took a few minutes but it did ensure that the core group was always consulted. Sometimes it was necessary to leave a copy of any planned documents (for example, drafts of assessment sheets or evaluation tools) for members to consider and discuss with colleagues outside the group. This method of approval was beneficial in encouraging all members of the PHC team to take part in the standard setting. The responsibility for ensuring that everyone was consulted was mine as facilitator. I also had the role of amending draft documents. Although I wrote up the documents, the contents were a team effort, each member having contributed opinions, information, research material or ideas.

The role of facilitator

I cannot overstress the importance of having a facilitator for the group. The facilitator's role is to organise meetings and to badger as many group members as possible into attending. Facilitators must ensure that all information is shared, that comments are collected and approval sought from absentees. They may have to delegate tasks to other group members and may have to negotiate differences of opinion on the wording used in the standards or audit documents. The facilitator must be a volunteer not a conscript, and should have the support of the team members when he/she has to negotiate, mediate and occasionally act as advocate for the less assertive members of the team who are sometimes overawed at practice meetings. The facilitator needs to be a skilled communicator and have a good understanding of group dynamics, if the group is to achieve its full potential. The facilitator may not necessarily be the same person for all the standard setting groups but should be identified at the outset. They have a key role in the productivity of the group and should be selected for their skills, not because they are the person with the most forceful manner, the loudest voice or the most authority in the practice.

The monitoring tools

Many more months of informal meetings and discussions, both in the practice and with others involved in standard setting in different areas, enabled us to complete the standard statement, determine the structure process and outcome criteria, and develop the monitoring tools. The monitoring tools comprised: (a) the clinic audit, an observation tool focusing on structural criteria such as the availability of health promotion material and accurate equipment in the clinic; (b) an audit tool for the clinic attenders' records; and (c) a questionnaire for clinic attenders (Gill, 1992).

Developing the monitoring tools proved to be the most difficult and time-consuming task, mainly because at the time there was no appropriate model. The team decided it must monitor criteria from each sector (structure, process and outcome) to pinpoint any failures.

Measuring outcomes alone would only indicate what had or had not been achieved and would not allow a full evaluation. A simple monitoring checklist was required which was easy to complete and which could be adapted for use in other clinics providing care for other groups within the practice population.

We also wanted to find out whether or not the people who attended the clinic were happy with the service being provided. Several pensioner clubs were visited to determine the wants of the potential clientele, and the following concerns about their visits to the health centre were identified:

- a lack of consideration regarding hearing defects or problems of mobility;
- staff were 'always in a rush';
- no time to explain tests, tablets or jargon.

Our concern was typified by the comment: 'I cannot bother the doctor with silly little things – although they are a worry'. Their expectations of the clinic were:

- it would provide an opportunity to ask the nurse or doctor about all health concerns, for example, swollen ankles, rashes, diet problems;
- they would have an 'MOT' (a health check-up);
- there would be time to discuss tablets, hospital tests and referrals;
- appointments would be convenient for people, fitting in with bus timetables or with appointments for spouses or friends.

These issues formed the basis of a questionnaire which we designed to assess the satisfaction of those who attended the clinic.

Monitoring the clinic

As with other major issues the actual method of monitoring the activities of the clinic was discussed with all members of the PHCT. Initially I suggested that the monitoring of the standards should be undertaken by a member of TCV staff who would be a neutral and unbiased observer. Some members expressed concern over maintaining confidentiality if an outside person was involved and so it was agreed that this should be carried out in house. In the normal course of events, practices do not have access to resources such as TCV. Other methods therefore have to be found to monitor standards. The solution in this case was that, to ensure a more objective view, staff not involved in running the clinic agreed to help me complete the audit checklists.

Monitoring of the clinic took place on two occasions using the observational audit tool. Clinic attenders' satisfaction questionnaires were completed by 30 people (approximately 17% of the attenders). A total of 180 records covering all attenders were examined.

I analysed the data from all the sources and found it to be both revealing and reassuring that time spent with the clinic attenders was of real benefit. The results of the monitoring activity are confidential to the practice and are not included here in detail. However, a comparison of the information on hospital discharge letters and the person's understanding of that consultation and the follow-up highlighted poor communication. There was also evidence of a lack of communication between hospital departments. The most significant point concerned patients' compliance with medication. Detailed discussion with patients revealed that the majority did not take their medication as prescribed.

On a more positive note, it was found that screening identified a variety of previously unreported diseases or disabilities, which were subsequently treated. These included six patients with hearing loss who had attributed this to the adverse effects of old age. 'It doesn't come on its own' was a frequent comment. The provision of a hearing aid greatly added to the quality of life for these patients.

Carers also were benefiting from the clinic. In one instance it was discovered that a family were at the end of their tether, trying to cope with a dementia sufferer. The family had not known that help was available until they brought their mother for her routine appointment at the clinic at which stage her condition, and that of her family, came to light.

Subsequent action

Analysis of the data was presented to the core team in a report which included my suggested solutions to the problems raised. These suggestions were all agreed and, where possible, implemented. However, with hindsight, I would not repeat this strategy. Instead, I would identify the problems but encourage the team to find their own solutions and to write their own action plans.

The team did develop an additional action plan for one major problem – maintaining privacy during consultations. Often staff had to interrupt a consultation to pass on the clinic attender's notes. A new system has since been introduced which involves clinic attenders taking responsibility for a queuing system and transporting their own notes from room to room. The difficulty of ensuring privacy and confidentiality occurred throughout all practice activities and it was decided that this needed further examination. Discussions resulted in the development of a practice protocol for maintaining confidentiality and privacy for patients. This now forms an integral part of practice procedures and this illustrates the effect of one audit exercise on other activities in a practice.

Other changes have taken place as a result of the audit. The concerns and expectations of clinic attenders have changed practice in the following ways:

- Nursing staff always discuss with a clinic attender their medication, hospital tests and referrals, and will refer to the GP if necessary, informing the GP of any proposed action.
- All staff do their best to ensure that the clinic attender understands their present health status; for example, their position on a waiting list.
- All staff demonstrate an awareness of the problems of hearing and mobility by seeking to ameliorate these conditions when possible.
- Staff operate a flexible appointment system within the allocated time and encourage people to drop in when necessary.
- Nursing staff will give 'flu vaccines and other prescribed injections during the clinic in order to save the attender having to make a return visit.
- To provide a more cost effective and efficient service, reception staff send copies of attenders' diagnostic test results with referral letters with the aim of reducing duplication of tests.
- There is an increased awareness of 'people-centredness' (WHPF, 1989) within the practice, demonstrated by the protocols (1) on repeat medication (providing a more efficient and effective service for the practice population, see Chapter 10) and (2) on privacy and confidentiality.
- A new assessment sheet used in the clinic facilitates a more holistic assessment of the attender's health status and needs. This document is also used for monitoring continuity of care and uniformity of advice.

Teamwork

As well as improving the quality of care of the practice population it was hoped that this collaborative approach would improve teamwork. Teamworking generally does improve when members spend time together but, given their present workload, members do not have time to undertake 'teamwork' for teamwork's sake, however desirable the concept. Nevertheless, this project demonstrated that time spent focusing attention on a practice activity such as the 'Well Elderly' clinic, one which is of concern to different disciplines, will improve many aspects of teamwork.

Frequent discussions (albeit often only very brief) brought about a better understanding within the team of their various roles. This improvement was not entirely due to the extra time spent together. The more important factor was how all concerned became aware that all were working towards a common goal, that is a better service for the older patient. Setting standards of care for their own and their colleagues' work places great emphasis on trust and value of opinions: if I am to work by your standards, I must trust your judgement and value your opinion and, if I am to set standards for your work, then I must trust you to work to the agreed standard. Conversely, you must trust me to do the same. Duplication of work can be avoided, but only if certain tasks can be delegated to others in the knowledge that they have the ability to perform the tasks to the standards which everyone has agreed.

Delegation and confidence in others' ability are the basic principles needed to set multidisciplinary standards of care and they build on a relationship of trust and value. Difficulties are bound to occur when trying to agree common goals and standards because team members have differing ideologies. PHC team members also have different boundaries of responsibility and it is often impossible to avoid 'treading on toes' (King's Fund Centre, 1990: 67). Specialist terminology used by different groups within the PHC team can also be a barrier to teamworking. Where abbreviations and jargon are used, it is important to be explicit and unambiguous so that everyone knows precisely what is meant. It is possible to overcome these difficulties, but it takes time because it requires an intimate understanding of the opinions and values of others. Time is one of the major problems with consensus standard setting but this project has found ways to overcome it. It is vital that as many PHC team members as possible attend an initial meeting to formulate plans for standard setting, so that everyone knows what is happening and so that the appropriate group can be selected. After the initial meeting, however, it is not essential for all members of the group to attend every meeting as long as they are consulted on all decisions.

Meeting together to set standards may reveal new resources available within the practice team. All members of PHCTs have contacts with a wide variety of people (Kestein & Savage, 1990). The contribution of the receptionists cannot be over-emphasised. Receptionists are usually local residents and, as such, know the facilities available and have an insight into the wants and needs of their community. This might be far more realistic than the views of other professionals who live or were brought up elsewhere, and it is valuable to include this local perspective in the planning of activities which are intended to raise the health of the practice population.

Conclusion

The alternative to a team setting its own standards is to follow the Dutch and US models and to have standards defined by those whose rationale may be expediency or cost control. The setting of national standards may be motivated by a number of different factors and may be less responsive to local community needs than standards set by the PHCT. Farmer (1991) suggests that many groups and organisations have an interest in influencing the care offered to patients. He advises that GPs should question the motives of, for example, hospital specialists who set policies which: 'fail to recognise fully the extent to which patients present their problems in different ways and vary in their response to, and expectations of, medical care.' (Farmer, 1991: 135)

This project has shown that a number of factors can contribute to the success of standard setting and auditing activities, including:

- the appointment of facilitators employed solely to assist PHCTs with these initiatives;
- the involvement of appropriate hospital consultants in standard setting teams, working with members of the PHCT;
- the full utilisation of the expertise already available amongst members of the PHCT;
- the utilisation of resources available in the local community, for example, schools for health promotion events, local colleges for printing artwork and business studies departments for skills in management;
- the utilisation of facilities in the community, for example, colleges can provide conference facilities and, on a smaller scale, are the ideal venue for workshops, seminars and postgraduate courses for team members;
- linking with local departments of nursing and medical education can provide teaching resources on this subject (see Chapters 6 and 12).

Setting multidisciplinary standards of care can provide us with the tools to critically examine and, more importantly, to evaluate the care which we provide for our patients as well as helping to engender teamworking amongst members of the PHCT. Irvine (1990:77) confidently states: 'practices which can show and justify the results of their work have nothing to fear from outside scrutiny because good results speak for themselves'.

References

DoH (1989) *Working for Patients*. HMSO, London.

Donabedian, A. (1966) Evaluating the quality of medical care. *Millbank Memorial Fund Quarterly*, **44**, 2, 166–206.

Farmer, A. (1991) Setting up of consensus standards for the care of patients in general practice. *British Journal of General Practice*, **41**, 135–6.

Gill, J. (1992) *Setting Multidisciplinary Standards of Care*. TCV Project Report. TCV, Welsh Office, Cardiff.

Irvine, D.H. (1990) Standards in general practice: the quality initiative revisited. *British Journal of General Practice*, February, 40, 75–7.

Kestein, J. & Savage, R. (1990) Geriatric screening in a rural practice: the financial implications. *British Journal of General Practice*, **40**, 513–15.

King's Fund Centre (1990) *Enhancing the Quality of Community Nursing*. King's Fund Centre, London.

Morison, M.J. (1992) Promoting the motivation to change. *Professional Nurse,* 7(11), 715–18.

Parsley, K. & Corrigan, P. (1994) *Quality Improvement in Nursing and Health Care. A Practical Approach.* Chapman & Hall, London.

RCGP (1985) *Policy Statement No. 2: Quality in General Practice.* November. Royal College of General Practitioners, London.

RCN (1990) *Quality Patient Care: The Dynamic Standard Setting System.* RCN, London.

Welsh Office (1990) *A Quality Health Service for Wales.* Welsh Office, Cardiff.

WHPF (1989) *Strategic Intent and Direction for the NHS in Wales.* Welsh Health Planning Forum, Cardiff.

Chapter 9

Valuing Interpersonal Skills in Health Visiting

Lisa Coles

There is a saying that 'what gets measured gets managed'. Health visitors are aware that much of their work that is aimed at promoting health is not fully recognised, given that evaluation of their work by managers is based on 'measured' or quantitative data (Kagan, 1985; Naish & Kline, 1990; Luker, 1992; Traynor, 1993). Much of their health promotion work involves the use of a range of interpersonal skills (IPSs). Ewles and Simnett (1992) have argued that health promotion will succeed or fail depending upon the effective use of IPSs. Simple performance indicators, such as the number and ages of clients seen and the proportion of children in a caseload that have received immunisation, do not reflect those activities which are hard to quantify, such as the use of IPSs.

Other community nurses may share this concern since health promotion is a required competency for all registered nurses (HMSO, 1983) and community health care nurses (UKCC, 1994). However, it is of particular relevance to health visitors as health promotion is fundamental to their practice. In my practice as a health visitor I work with colleagues who demonstrate the skills of health promotion and IPSs daily. The question is: how can this process information be captured in measuring health visitor intervention?

The concept of interpersonal skill

IPSs in the nursing field in general refer to the social and emotional features of care rather than to manual and technical features (Kagan, 1985). Dickson *et al.* (1989) have defined IPSs as a series of appropriate, co-ordinated and integrated non-verbal and verbal interactions which have as their purpose the achievement of a particular goal.

The literature on IPSs offers some theoretical approaches, including:

- the technological or mechanical nature of using IPSs (Argyle, 1982);
- the goal directedness of skill usage (Crute *et al.*, 1989);
- the intentions of certain interventions (Heron, 1986);
- the use of IPSs in problem solving (Egan, 1990);
- the therapeutic and client centredness of IPSs (Rogers & Stevens, 1967).

Two particular features of IPSs usage identified in the literature are the cognitive aspect (knowing which behaviours are appropriate given certain interactional goals), and the caring or affective aspects (perceiving the feelings of the other person, being non-judgmental, praising the client's progress and befriending) (Burnard, 1989; Ewles & Simnett, 1992). Kagan (1985) argues that the decision about which skills to use in specific contexts of practice is more crucial than the performance of these skills.

The general aim of health promotion is that of improving health and developing control over it (Downie *et al.*, 1990; Ewles & Simnett, 1992). Within this broad remit, Ewles and Simnett describe the aims and values of five different approaches to health promotion:

- the medical;
- the behavioural;
- the educational;
- the societal;
- the client centred.

The last of these includes enabling and empowering clients to take health improving action.

The project

In reviewing the literature and in considering these 'less tangible skills' of health visiting, it became apparent that they will always be difficult to measure or direct as a resource, unless they are first identified by a common nomenclature, and can be evaluated in practice.

Having identified this practice issue I realised that I would not have the time in my work as a health visitor to investigate it further and it was at this point that I discussed the project with my nurse manager and TCV. I was appointed as a short-term clinical fellow with TCV for one session per week for two years and my nurse manager was able to match this time, enabling me to undertake the project and register for the degree of Master of Philosophy/Doctorate at the University of Wales College of Medicine.

The aim of the project was to test the proposition that a skills-focused approach to analysing health promotion activities might lead to a means of expressing this less measurable aspect of health visiting (Coles, 1993). In the following discussion the process of data collection and some data from the health visitors and clients is presented followed by a consideration of the relationship between IPSs and outcomes of care.

The health visitors' study

I first researched whether and how IPSs are used by health visitors to promote health. My aim was to generate a taxonomy of IPSs used in this context. I used the critical incident technique (Flanagan, 1954) to find out which IPSs are practised by health visitors.

All the health visitors in one health unit were asked to describe in writing an interaction with a client or clients which had involved health promotion, one where they felt they had used IPSs effectively. The terms 'IPSs' and 'health promotion' were not defined, because I wanted a definition grounded in practice to emerge from the words and phrases used by the health visitors themselves.

The critical incidents reported most frequently were parents with emotional health and relationship needs of their own, and babies and toddlers with nutritional and behaviour difficulties. In both cases, problems were often interlinked, complex and multidimensional, reflecting the broad definition of health with which health visitors work.

A content analysis of the narratives generated a classification of the interpersonal skills used in practice. Their process of use, their special attributes such as caring and cognitive skills, and their related characteristics such as personal qualities and broad approaches, were separately categorised. This classification has resulted in a list of IPSs used by this sample of health visitors (Table 9.1).

Three of these – listening, paraphrasing and questioning – are basic communication skills. Non-verbal behaviour was the second most frequent skill that the respondents were aware of using and of observing in others. It encompassed phrases such as 'using touch to demonstrate care'. Communicating facts, the third most frequently recorded activity, indicates a more educational approach to health promotion.

The remaining skills of valuing and accepting, helping people talk, forming strategies, facilitating autonomy, befriending, empathising, and promoting positive feelings, all contribute to a picture of a client-centred health promotion model, that is one of empowering and enabling clients to progress towards health goals achievable within their own life context (Ewles & Simnett, 1992).

Each heading in Table 9.1 is the result of grouping words and phrases into categories. Helping people talk, for example, is the

Table 9.1 Taxonomy of IPSs used by health visitors ranked according to frequency of use

	Frequency of use
Listening	17
Non-verbal behaviour	14
Communicating facts	12
Valuing and accepting	9
Helping people talk	8
Forming strategies	7
Facilitating autonomy	6
Befriending	4
Empathising	4
Promoting positive feelings	4
Paraphrasing	2
Questioning	2

heading for a number of responses about allowing clients time and space to explore and express their feelings.

One independent reviewer questioned whether or not 'befriending' was a skill. In the analysis, it was included as a skill if, in the context of its use in the critical incident, it appeared to be the conscious intention of the health visitor to befriend the client for a particular purpose rather than just to adopt a friendly manner or approach.

In describing an incident many of the respondents offered an evaluation of their work when summarising their health promotion objectives. These showed that short-term, structured objectives were easiest for them to evaluate and that broad, long-term objectives were the most difficult.

The clients' study

The health visitors' study on its own would provide a one-sided view of IPSs, resting as it does on health visitors' interpretations of the skills that they used. To obtain a different perspective on the work of health visitors and their skills, a guided interview schedule was designed, and in-depth interviews were undertaken with the clients of health visitors. The aim was to obtain an evaluation of the health visitors' IPSs by some users of the service. In addition, comments were sought on the effectiveness of health visitor interventions.

An initial analysis of the transcripts of the taped interviews showed that the clients recognised many of the skills the health visitors themselves had identified; especially 'befriending' and 'helping people talk' by giving them time. Also of importance to clients were continuity of care by the same health visitor (sometimes over many years and involving other members of the family), ready access, and availability for home visits.

Clients also gave examples of inadequate IPSs which confirmed the importance of health visitors 'getting it right' from the clients' perspective. Criticism was made, for example, of rushed attention:

> 'I didn't feel there was any rapport there. I don't feel she was genuinely, genuinely interested in me. I just feel I was one of a number going in and out. You know, strip the baby off, get the baby weighed, any questions, OK off you go.'

The same mother contrasted this with her contact with another health visitor:

> 'I was in tears on the 'phone, so up she came and she just sat down and talked to me. She was there in ten minutes and she talked, she was with me. What I liked about her was she wasn't rushed, she sat down, she had plenty of time for me. She didn't make me feel like an idiot, though I did feel it, and she watched me breast feed, she watched me latch the baby on. She had time to stay. She was just wonderful. She was like a friend as well you know, always at the end of the 'phone. She didn't seem to think anything would be too much trouble. She made my life easier and gave me confidence.'

The clients emphasised personal health matters in their interviews, indicating a broader range of concerns than emerged in the health visitor study. These included, for example, children with chronic illness and disability. To assess the effectiveness of interventions in relation to change in their knowledge, attitudes or behaviours clients were able to identify critical incidents. These assessments involved a value judgement identifying some 'good' which had come from the incident.

In relation to their contact with health visitors it was not difficult for clients to describe the benefits. Mary, for example, described her change in attitude and behaviour:

> 'I can remember when she went. I said: "Thank God she'd come to see me today" because she did change my whole attitude, you know, and I think baby is a better sleeper because of it.... I put into practice what she showed me could work.'

There were several additional health gains from this one incident:

- Mary's mother felt she 'had learnt something new' about child care.
- Mary's husband no longer 'walked the boards' with the crying baby at night.
- Their toddler who was 'more involved' with the baby's care.
- The two friends who had picked up useful information from what Mary had learnt from the health visitor.

- Mary's increased confidence: 'I cope on my own now'.
- Mary's change in her attitude to her own body once successful breast feeding was established.

Discussion

For many of the aims of health visiting it is not possible to calculate a rate of successful outcomes. For example, one of the health gain targets set by the Welsh Health Planning Forum (1993) is to promote the development of confident and caring parents. It is not that the target is wrong or that achievement of such an aim is not already common in health visiting. How do you know if the intervention of health visitors and other health professionals are contributing to the achievement of this target? What is a confident or caring parent? It therefore seems inappropriate to think only in terms of measurement of outcomes. It is difficult to predict outcomes against which to measure interventions since the expected number of parents in a given caseload or practice who do not fulfil such a definition is unknown. A parent may be confident or caring with one child but not with another, and may be confident and caring one moment and then not at another when, for example, under additional stress. Any figure purporting to measure the confidence and care of parents will have little real meaning. In contrast, it is quite clear what is meant by a 95% uptake of immunisation against whooping cough of all children born in a certain year.

There is also the problem of evaluating outcomes that are not related to national health gain targets (WHPF, 1989; DoH, 1992). The pursuit of national targets, such as those relating to immunisation, can reduce the time given to the local and individual search for other health needs, one of the four principles of health visiting (Council for the Education and Training of Health Visitors, 1982). Rather a two-way process is desirable in which practitioners inform practice colleagues, commissioners and managers, when they find additional, and possibly more pressing, local health needs. This process should lead to the occasional revision of service targets.

Egan (1990) argues that the process of using skills is often as valuable as the outcome. Process and outcome should be considered separately, distinguishing the use of appropriate clinical activity (including IPSs) as a process measure, and of health gain (linked to practice protocols and local strategic targets) as an outcome measure. Employing the qualitative research and evaluation methods used in the field of education (Miles & Huberman, 1994), and the qualitative research methods used alongside quantitative methods in nursing research (Corner 1991), may prove more productive in evaluating the process of health visiting.

The process and appropriateness of clinical activity can be assessed, for example, by clinical supervision. Clinical supervision, although not fully developed in community health care nursing (Bishop, 1994), may prove to be a suitable way of formalising expertise in the use of IPSs for health promotion. The use of critical incidents (as in this project) in clinical supervision may help to develop skills in precise observation, by promoting more accurate description and by discouraging assumptions about clients' and practitioners' behaviours.

Health gain as an outcome measure is problematic in several ways. The client needs to be involved both in defining expected outcomes and in reviewing outcomes following intervention. Questions need to be asked of the client: before the intervention to set the criteria for success, and after the intervention to describe health gain. For example:

- After you talked with the health visitor can you say if you or your family had gained anything?
- In what way were you helped regarding the matter you were talking about?
- Have you since done anything differently or made any changes?
- Do you think differently now about the matter you talked about?

If it is necessary to seek to attribute the outcome to a particular practitioner's intervention an additional question could be asked: could any other member of the primary health care team do for this client what this health visitor (or other practitioner) is doing?

The concept of causal links is a philosophical one and difficult to define (Miles & Huberman, 1994). A direct causal link between specific interpersonal intervention and health gain was not possible to identify from either set of research data. But, on occasions, particularly when drawing upon the testimony of clients, it was possible to be confident that intervention had had a positive impact.

The health visitors' accounts of their use of IPSs in day-to-day health promoting events allowed me both to compile a taxonomy of IPSs and to examine the context in which such skills are used. The interviews with clients confirmed the use of several of the skills the health visitors had identified. These can be more fully understood when the client's perception is added. For example, when I enquired further about a statement from a client that 'she was like a friend' it became apparent that 'befriending' is associated with: loyalty, trust, support, concern, giving sound advice, being there and helping plan.

Together, both studies refute the assumption that IPSs are invisible, or lacking in tangibility. IPSs are apparent to practitioners and users in a way that is relevant to their concerns about their own and their families' health. These skills are not invisible as far as these health visitors and clients are concerned.

References

Argyle, M. (1982) *The Psychology of Interpersonal Behaviour.* Penguin, Harmondsworth.

Bishop, V. (1994) Clinical supervision for an accountable profession. *Nursing Times*, **90**(39), 35–7.

Burnard, P. (1989) *Therapy in Practice, 10: Teaching Interpersonal Skills*. Chapman & Hall, London.

Coles, L. (1993) *Health Visitors' Interpersonal Skills for Health Promotion*. TCV Report. TCV, Welsh Office, Cardiff.

Corner, J. (1991) In search of more complete answers to research questions. Quantitative versus qualitative research methods: is there a way forward? *Journal of Advanced Nursing*, **16**(6), 718–27.

Council for the Education and Training of Health Visitors (1982) *Health Visiting: Principles in Practice*. Council for the Education and Training of Health Visitors, London.

Crute, V.C., Hargie, O.D.W. & Ellis, R.A.F. (1989) An evaluation of a communication skills course for health visitor students. *Journal of Advanced Nursing*, **14**(7), 546–52.

Dickson, D.A., Hargie, O.D.W. & Morrow, N.C. (1989) *Communication Skills Training for Health Professionals*. Chapman & Hall, London.

DoH (1992) *The Health of the Nation: A Strategy for Health in England*. HMSO, London.

Downie, R.S., Fyfe, C. & Tannahill, A. (1990) *Health Promotion Models and Values*. Oxford University Press, Oxford.

Egan, G. (1990) *The Skilled Helper: A Systematic Approach to Effective Helping*, 4th edn. Thompson Information. Publishing Group, Brack/Cole Publishing Co., Pacific Grove, California.

Ewles, L. & Simnett, I. (1992) *Promoting Health: A Practical Guide*, 2nd edn. Scutari Press, London.

Flanagan, J. (1954) The critical incident technique. *Psychological Bulletin*, **51**, 327–58.

Heron, J. (1986) *Six Category Intervention Analysis*, 2nd edn. Human Potential Research Project, University of Surrey, Guildford.

HMSO (1983) *Nurses, Midwives and Health Visitors Approval Order*. HMSO, London.

Kagan, C. (ed.) (1985) *Interpersonal Skills in Nursing: Research and Applications*. Croom Helm, Sydney.

Luker, K.A. (1992) Evaluating practice. In: *Health Visiting: Towards Community Health Nursing*, K.A. Luker and J. Orr (eds), Chapter 5, 159-90. Blackwell Science, Oxford.

Miles, M.B. & Huberman, A.M. (1994) *Qualitative Data Analysis: An Expanded Source Book*, 2nd edn. Sage Publications, Thousand Oaks.

Naish, K. & Kline, R. (1990) What counts can't always be counted. *Health Visitor*, **63**(12), 421–2.

Rogers, C.R. & Stevens, B. (1967) *Person to Person: The Problem of Being Human*. Real People Press, Lafayette, California.

Traynor, M. (1993) Some current issues for health visiting. *Health Visitor*, **66**(6), 216–18.

UKCC (1994) *The Future of Professional Practice – The Council's Standards for Education and Practice following Registration*. UKCC, London.

WHPF (1989) *The Strategic Intent and Direction for the NHS in Wales*. Welsh Office, Cardiff.

WHPF (1993) *Health and Social Gain for Children: Guidance to Inform Local Strategies for Health*. Welsh Office, Cardiff.

Chapter 10

Changing Prescribing Practices

Carl Venn

To understand the development of this project, it is helpful if I begin with a short autobiographical introduction. I was born and bred in South Wales but, although I travelled only as far as Bristol to train, it had never really been in my mind to return to the town of my birth to work there as a GP. However, after my house-jobs, I returned to the Valleys to do my vocational training in the Rhondda, based at East Glamorgan General Hospital.

In 1990, Dr Colin Dexter, a close friend and fellow trainee at East Glamorgan, invited me to join his single-handed practice in a small town in the eastern Valleys as a part-time partner. The offer was not an easy one to accept as the town was where my father had been born and brought up and it was deeply engrained in me that one moved from rather than to the Valleys. Although I was reluctant to return to the Valleys, the prospect of working in a small team and with a stable population proved to be irresistible and I joined the practice in August of 1990.

As I was part-time with the practice and at that stage we did not anticipate rapid expansion, I began to look around for alternative employment for the other sessions. I heard about TCV and about the positions being advertised of clinical fellow. It sounded ideal, providing academic stimulation and opportunities to explore the medical services of the Valleys with a broader eye than our small practice could provide. I also felt that I would have something to offer the project, being a GP concurrently providing PHC in the TCV target area. I applied and was appointed as one of two half-time clinical fellows in September 1990.

Very early on, the clinical fellows decided to flee the TCV offices in Cardiff and get out among the Valley practices. This was the steep part of our learning curve. We met many grassroots PHC workers and found out about some of the local initiatives which they were already undertaking. We heard about problem areas and the difficulties which they were facing, and the ways in which they were or were not coping.

Continuing medication

From this initial contact with the practices I developed a particular interest in the organisation and practice of continuing medication. This fascinating multidisciplinary interface became the specific area of my work within TCV. My interest initially focused on the potential value for patients of attending a continuing medication clinic (Venn, 1991). This idea originated with Dr Dare, a practitioner in the area. He felt that there were in most practices, even the smallest ones, a number of patients with conditions where close monitoring of therapy was advisable. He mentioned people suffering from epilepsy, thyroid disease, and those using drugs like Lithium and Digoxin where the therapeutic margin was narrow.

With his co-operation, one of his practice nurses and I set up a 'Continuing Medication Clinic' in his practice as a pilot study. Patients attending the clinic received education on their medication as well as an assessment of their level of understanding, measurement of certain physical parameters and, where appropriate, blood tests.

Sadly the FHSA was not willing to fund the clinic as an ongoing concern and so it was not possible to continue with it, despite the fact that the screening that we had carried out had identified individuals with a variety of problems including over- and under-treatment.

Repeat prescribing

Running the clinic, however, opened my eyes to deficiencies in the way repeat prescribing was working in my own practice. My interest thus shifted from continuing medication to the area of repeat prescribing. Interestingly repeat prescribing was not mentioned as a problem area in the visits that the clinical fellows had made the previous year.

Like many practices in the Valleys, ours was small. Our repeat prescribing system (RPS), such as it was at that time, was extremely patient-friendly. It was not computerised. A patient requested their drugs, either directly or via a variety of intermediaries, and then waited as the receptionist took out the notes. She checked that the drugs had been issued before and, if they had, she then wrote out the prescription and presented it to be signed by the GP. The GP signed this between seeing patients in surgery. The receptionist then entered the issue in the patient's notes. If there was a question about the medication, this was put to the doctor when the script was given to him together with the patient's notes for his perusal.

Subsequent experience has taught me that this kind of RPS is very common in practices in the TCV area. As I examined the system we had in place, and considered alternatives and ways of improving it, I learned two important and fairly obvious lessons:

- Properly planned RPSs can look complex but they share the important characteristic that they can be thoroughly examined and audited.
- No matter what the system is, it can almost certainly be improved.

These two lessons have been confirmed by every investigation I have subsequently carried out. Having looked at our RPS, I began to talk about changing it. At this point I learned a third lesson – there are always many reasons put forward to discourage change:

- 'The patients will not put up with it.'
- 'They will leave the practice and go to others who prescribe more easily.'
- 'They will never be able to learn new ways.'

These arguments were not only put to me by the reception staff but, when I discussed my plans with other doctors, some too were equally discouraging.

Nevertheless we persevered and drew up proposals for our new system. We informed all the patients receiving repeat prescriptions that the system would be changed, how and why, and we told them when the changes would occur and what would be expected of them.

When the change occurred none of the prophecies of doom were realised, and the problems generated by the system have been negligible. This produced two more important lessons:

- Changes to RPSs need not be large and revolutionary to produce significant benefits.
- Change need not be painful if it is planned well.

Auditing repeat prescribing systems

This work in my own practice was done in my own time, but I began to see an application for it in my work with TCV. It seemed to me that there was a place for someone who could help and advise practices about their repeat prescribing systems. Someone who could help them prevent waste, improve record-keeping, check compliance, avoid abuse and generally improve the efficiency of this part of their practice. Medications are an expensive part of the overall medical budget and repeat prescriptions make up the bulk of this. It would surely be worthwhile to look into initiatives which would help ensure that only necessary medicines were supplied under RPSs.

I spoke about these ideas to Dr. Fuge, who was the Regional Medical Officer to the Welsh Office at this time and who was seconded on a one day a week basis to the Gwent FHSA as an Independent Medical Advisor in the field of prescribing issues. She was often called to visit practices where there were problems with drug costs and she agreed that sometimes the RPSs were inadequate. All she herself could do, however, was to threaten or cajole, but now I was offering her the possibility of a helping hand, someone who could spend some time facilitating change in these practices.

Following this conversation, I was contacted by a local practice where there were considerable problems with the RPS. The practice had received several visits from Dr. Fuge and were very keen to do all that they could to improve their poor performance. Over the next eighteen months I became very closely involved with this practice, working with the staff to audit the system and to reconstruct it on more efficient lines.

The first phase was the assessment of the problem. For this, I conducted a simple audit of 100 repeat prescription requests. I sat in the reception area and observed how these requests were delivered and how they were dealt with. Later I reviewed the notes to determine their quality.

I can honestly say that this was one of the most eye-opening experiences of my life. It made me realise that, as GPs, we are protected by our reception staff from raw exposure to the general public. Patients arriving in our consultation rooms have already been 'processed' a little by the staff. The patients' expectations, their ideas, have been affected by their brief encounters with 'the girls on the desk'. As I sat and listened to encounter after encounter, I felt humbled at the realisation of how much unscrambling of needs goes on before the door of the GP's room opens. Perhaps this practice was exceptional in degree but, subsequently, similar experience has shown me that it was not unusual in kind.

After this initial audit had been completed, a programme of action was instituted. It was agreed that it was necessary to establish a database in the first instance which recorded which patients were receiving what drugs. This required the reception staff through their contacts with patients to distribute a questionnaire. The staff were fully co-operative until it was discovered that the extra work they were undertaking would not be funded by the practice. There were background problems which had produced resentment and frustration and things came to a head at this point. The collection of data continued but at a much reduced level and eventually at such a low level that the project could not continue. Despite my efforts to maintain a momentum, I was forced to withdraw. All the practice appeared to have gained at this stage was written proof that things needed to improve. The work, however, was not completely forgotten and the practice has subsequently undergone some revolutionary changes which will hopefully lead to permanent improvements.

During this time I also visited other practices in the area and conducted audits of their RPSs. It was necessary in each case to visit the practice on several occasions. I used the first visit to meet the staff and to gain their confidence. Having an outsider coming in to audit your work can be threatening, especially if you are a receptionist and the outsider is a doctor. So I tried hard to get to know the staff and the system thoroughly. If possible on this visit, I would sit to watch through a surgery – at the desk, to see the RPS in action. Often how it was described and how it was implemented in practice were quite different.

Having carried out these initial observations, I would design an audit appropriate for that practice. As each practice is different, and each RPS has evolved under different constraints, I did not find it helpful to develop just one all-purpose audit, but rather to tailor each investigation to the individual system. The questions I sought to answer were, however, broadly the same:

- How busy is the system?
- How good is the record keeping?
- How efficient is the system by its own standards?
- How are problems dealt with?
- Is the system used to maximum effect and, in particular, does it pick up non-compliance or abuse?

Following the audit, I prepared a report which reduced the data collected to important practical issues. I then returned with this to the practice, along with suggestions on how the system might be improved and commendation on its strong points. In some cases, practices instituted changes and I was called back to repeat the audit some time later to monitor improvements.

During my time at TCV, our practice expanded by the assimilation of another list. Eventually, increasing demands there meant that my contract with TCV had to come to an end and I became a full-time GP.

Just prior to leaving TCV, however, there was a further interesting development. It involved a group of practices in the area who were cooperating together on an on-call rota. They were eager to develop a common strategy across practice boundaries, for a number of core activities including repeat prescribing.

For this local initiative I prepared a document outlining minimum standards in repeat prescribing, and the practices undertook the audit outlined above. The plan is to move all the participating practices towards agreed standards for their RPSs. Sadly, with all the changes in general practice being implemented at the moment, this project is losing priority.

Conclusion

What then are my thoughts reflecting back on this project? I thoroughly enjoyed the three years with TCV and personally gained much from the experience. I met many interesting professionals and came across a variety of initiatives and points of view which I would have missed had I not joined the project. My biggest regret is that TCV lasted such a short time. As a GP still practising in the area, I very much miss the resource of TCV and the stimulation it provided. It seemed to disappear without replacement just as it was gaining credibility and acceptance.

As far as my work in the field of repeat prescribing is concerned, I still feel that there is much to be done. I am not aware that any help is being made available to practices that wish to improve the safety and efficiency of their RPSs. Without such help, a large proportion of the resources currently being placed into the promotion of rational prescribing will fail to have the desired impact, particularly in regard to costs.

Reference

Venn, C. (1991) *Continuing medication in the community – is it a problem?* TCV Discussion Paper 7. TCV, Welsh Office, Cardiff.

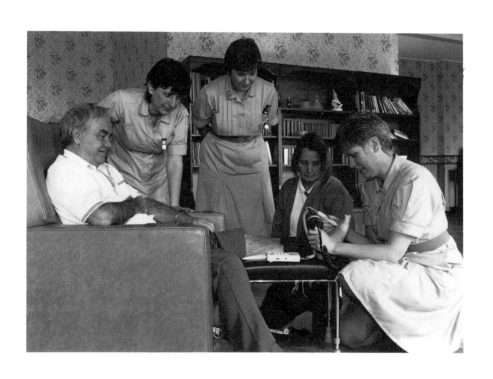

Section 3

Education

The quality of PHC is fundamentally influenced by the educational preparation of, and subsequent support for, PHC practitioners. Much care in the community is provided by individual practitioners or small groups. In part, they are the gatekeepers to more specialised health care and this requires up-to-date knowledge and skills (as argued earlier in Chapters 6, 7 and 10). Their isolation from educational centres and pressure upon their time, however, may restrict their opportunities for such development.

Brian Wallace, in the TCV Strategy Document (Teamcare Valleys, 1990), referred to the observation of Lord Rosenheim, two decades ago, that the health of the population could be 'vastly improved' if only current medical knowledge was fully applied. Hart (1988) similarly noted that the findings of medical science were not being applied in general practice, especially in the areas of prevention, screening of high-risk patients, and the care of chronic illness. The emphasis on 'evidence-based practice' which is now a priority of the health service agenda is the latest manifestation of this concern.

This section includes four chapters that focus on the need for training and education, and on how this might best be met. At one level the objective is to tackle ignorance and to disseminate up-to-date knowledge. At another it is to help practitioners gain a better understanding of what they are doing and of their strengths and weaknesses.

There has been a massive expansion in the number of nurses employed in practices. What are their current needs for education and training? How can their role within PHC be best served by the provision of in-service training opportunities? Chapter 11 draws upon a survey of all practice nurses in the TCV area. It pays particular attention to their contribution in health promotion and the prevention of disease. What the survey reveals is that this is a group of nurses who have been poorly prepared for their current roles.

There are statutory requirements upon doctors (through the PGEA) and on nurses (through PREPP) to undertake in-service training. Many PHC professionals however are working in isolated communities, under heavy workloads and distant from centres of professional education. For them distance learning opportunities may be the best way of gaining education, but at present these are very limited. Through assessing educational needs in the area, TCV developed and tested a distinctive strategy: one based on needs assessment, piloting, auditing and testing. Chapter 12 details a case study: the development, production and provision of a course on ophthalmology in general practice.

Practitioners are well placed to undertake research. As PHC professionals, doctors and nurses are expected to be involved in research. What problems might they face, however, when attempting to study what they actually do in practice? Particularly at a time when there are important national policy discussions about changes in the duties and responsibilities of a particular group, it is important that these deliberations should be informed by good and sensitive research. Should members of such a group undertake this research, or is it best left to more detached researchers with no specific experience of that practice in that particular area? How should they draw upon their clinical experience and knowledge? Chapter 13 reports on some of the problems that practitioners face when they take on such research and acquire the identity of 'researcher'.

There is widespread ignorance in PHC about certain areas of important but unfashionable health care. One such area is the treatment of venous ulcers. Chapter 14 reports upon a study which examined the training, role and knowledge of GPs, practice nurses and district nurses, concerning the care of patients with venous ulcers. Also it reports upon an audit of medical and nursing records. What it found was an alarming level of ignorance not just about diagnosis and treatment but also about patient education.

The chapters in this section demonstrate the critical importance of training and education. Levels of ignorance and expressed educational need warrant major investment in this area. The policy of appointing practitioners to clinical fellowships is one option which we would advocate. As the experience of TCV clearly demonstrates, clinical fellows were able to develop the knowledge base needed for their practice while remaining in, or in close touch with, practice. Moreover by working within the local area they were able to contribute directly to the knowledge base of others.

What this section also does is raise fundamental questions about what a particular group of practitioners actually do – in practice, in reality, not in theory – and how their present contribution to the work of the PHCT might be strengthened and developed. Striving to understand what it is that we are doing is, arguably, a fundamental goal of applied education and an issue of increasing importance as professional boundaries become less rigid.

References

Hart, J.T. (1988) *A New Kind of Doctor*. Merlin Press, London.
Teamcare Valleys (1990) *Strategy Document*. TCV, Welsh Office, Cardiff.

Chapter 11

Identifying the Training Needs of Practice Nurses

Gwen Davies

More than half of all the NHS staff are nurses and nearly a quarter of all health service expenditure is directed at nursing (UKCC, 1986). These facts have great relevance to the shape, quality and cost of health care as a whole. Of all the qualified nurses employed in the NHS, more than half work outside the hospital setting (UKCC, 1986). Despite this, there has been little or no discussion by policy makers outside nursing about the organisation, management and future direction of nursing practice. If we are to improve the health of the nation, the government needs to look at what nurses have to offer. They are a large workforce and, with properly directed training, they could have a huge impact on improving the health of the population.

The introduction of the 1990 GP Contract produced changes in the practice and reimbursement of fees for GPs. It also brought about many changes in the delivery of PHC services. One such change was an increase in the number of practice nurses employed by GPs. Many new practice nurses were employed, primarily to assist with the implementation of the extra work that the Contract brought to general practice.

Prior to the increase in the employment of practice nurses, there had been little consultation between DHAs, FHSAs and GPs, about the services that were already being offered and about those that could be developed by other nursing disciplines working in the community. The numbers of practice nurses were increased with little thought being given, or research undertaken, into the needs of the population, or into the services these nurses could effectively develop to improve the population's health.

The study

This chapter describes some of the findings which emerged from a study I undertook while working at TCV as a full-time clinical fellow (Davies, 1993). This focused on the role and training needs of practice nurses. Particular attention is given at the end of the chapter to their need for training regarding health promotion and the prevention of disease.

A comprehensive literature review enabled me to assess what work had already been carried out in this field. This revealed that little comparable research had been undertaken. I did learn, however, of a national study then being carried out by the Social Policy Research Unit, University of York, and I visited the researchers there to learn more about their survey which has since been published (Atkin *et al.*, 1993). This preparatory work assisted me with the design of a self-completion postal questionnaire.

For nursing research to be useful, it must speak to practising nurses and, in planning the study, it was important that I was aware of the conditions of work, the routines and the concerns of practice nurses. To this end, I studied the work of one practice nurse. I worked with her as a participant observer over a period of three months. This was a rewarding experience as it revealed the extent of the experience and training she needed to carry out the demanding work that was expected of her. During this period my interests became more structured, helping me decide what questions should be included in the questionnaire. The benefit of being a participant observer was that by questioning why and how certain procedures were carried out, and through observing her at work, I gained a clearer understanding of the work of practice nurses.

The sample

The intention of the research was to distribute the questionnaire to all practice nurses who were working in general practices in the TCV area. For this study no differentiation was made according to the qualifications they held. A practice nurse was considered to be either a State Registered Nurse (SRN/RGN) or a State Enrolled Nurse (SEN/EN) who was working as a 'practice nurse' in a general practice.

I had assumed that a comprehensive list would be available through the five FHSAs that covered the TCV area. However, when I came to distributing the questionnaires, I found this information was not available. Compiling a list from scratch was time-consuming and involved me in a great deal of liaison and consultation, both with staff working in general practices and with the PHC facilitators based in the five FHSAs. As a result of these enquiries I was able to produce a list of 232 practice nurses.

The questionnaire

A 22-page questionnaire including both open and closed questions was piloted with four practice nurses working outside the TCV area and on two nurse colleagues in TCV. As expected, the questionnaire needed to be modified to remove certain ambiguities. The questionnaire included questions on:

- personal and employment details;
- qualifications and experience;
- training obtained and desired on a range of topics;
- access to training and professional advice and support;
- teamwork within the PHCT;
- extent and variety of work undertaken;
- attitudes to changes since implementation of the 1990 GP Contract.

During June 1992, I sent the questionnaires out with a covering letter to all the practice nurses who I had identified as working in the TCV area. Confidentiality was guaranteed and participants were asked to return the questionnaire to TCV in an enclosed Freepost envelope. A letter of explanation was also sent to FHSA managers and to GPs.

In the first four weeks I received only 57 returned questionnaires. Non-responders were sent a reminder. This produced a further 30 responses. A final follow-up was carried out by telephone. It was only then that I began to discover the extent of the inaccuracies in the database I had prepared. For example, I found that five of the practice nurses had received duplicate questionnaires. As they worked in both main and branch surgeries, their names had been included twice on the database. Another surgery employed only one practice nurse but had been sent four questionnaires. This was because, when compiling the database, I had been given the names of her two predecessors and both her single and married names. In other instances, although nurses were no longer employed in a practice, their names had been passed on to me. Through these contacts, I was able to reduce the list of eligible practice nurses from 232 names to 210.

The overall number who eventually returned a completed questionnaire was 100 (48%). It is probable that many of those who failed to respond were working under considerable pressure and felt they simply did not have the time to complete the questionnaire.

Some findings

Who practice nurses are and what they do

A total of 60 of the sample were first appointed as practice nurses during the three years from September 1989, a few months prior to the introduction of the GP Contract in April 1990. Table 11.1 compares

Table 11.1 Practice nurses: age by length of appointment

Age	Length of appointment	
	Up to 3 years	More than 3 years
21–30	21	2
31–40	17	11
41–50	13	17
50+	9	10
Total	60	40

their age distribution with that of those who had been appointed before September 1989.

Bolden and Takle (1984) and Stilwell and Drury (1988) both found in their studies that practice nurses were mainly aged 35 years and over. My survey however suggests that practice nursing is now attracting nurses in the younger age groups. This could be due, as one practice nurse suggested, to the belief that:

> 'Practice nursing is now a definite career choice for not only nurses with children, but also those who wish to pursue a career. It lets them develop fully as a specialised practitioner.... Now is the time to make practice nursing a choice that has the same professional status and recognition as district nursing and health visiting.'

Most of the respondents were employed to work as 'practice nurses' only. Sixteen, however, were employed to undertake other jobs such as receptionist and practice manager. One nurse described the duties expected of her as follows: 'I have to take out and re-file patients' notes, answer the telephone, write repeat prescriptions, take house calls, deal with hospital appointments, book ambulances, and deal with referral letters.'

Another said she was responsible for: 'organising the pay and FHSA returns, co-ordinating 'flu injection programmes in early autumn, and arranging education from reps.'

Only one in five of the respondents had a full-time contract of 37.5 hours. Four out of five worked part-time with the weekly hours ranging from 6 to 36 hours. The mean hours worked was 25.5 hours.

Training

The experience and training that the practice nurses brought with them to general practice varied considerably. This study found that 77 had received all their previous experience in hospitals. Only 23 of the nurses had any community training prior to becoming a practice nurse. Of these 23, 16 had been given training on a practice nurse course, and seven had a district nursing qualification – two of these seven also had a health visiting qualification.

The main obstacle reported by the respondents preventing them obtaining further training was the lack of staff cover. Nearly half gave this reason. Under the 1990 Contract, GPs are required to provide opportunities for their employees to obtain appropriate education and training. The nurses are put in a difficult position by not being offered relevant training for the job in hand: to improve the health status of their practice population. As one practice nurse wrote in her questionnaire: 'I would like to see a more formal and comprehensive course before taking up the post. I often feel thrown in at the deep end and am expected to muddle through'.

Another stated: 'I do feel very strongly that this is a demanding job and that nurses should have a wide experience before taking up a position in practice nursing.'

Knowledge and training in health promotion

Many practice nurses are employed mainly to undertake health promotion work delegated to them by their GPs. Their knowledge and training on how to manage health promotion clinics, how to make health promotion effective, and how to improve the health status of the practice population, is important.

When asked what training they had received on how to manage health promotion clinics, 81 responded. Of these, 19% had received no training, 26% had been given training only by their GP, 2% had been trained during their basic nurse training, 32% on a local course, and 21% said they had received training from another source such as journals, books, drug representatives and other nurses. Overall 31% felt a need for further training.

A total of 92 responded to the question: 'Have you received training on how to make health promotion effective?'. Of these, 42% said they had received no training. The source of training of those who said they had received training was: 5% during their basic nurse training, 16% by their GPs, 25% on a local course and 12% from another source. Overall 26% felt a need for more training.

When asked if they had been given any training on how to improve the health status of the practice population, 91 responded to this question. A total of 69% said they had received no training and 33% felt a need for further training.

These findings show that on average between a quarter and a third of the practice nurses who responded felt that they were inadequately trained in specific areas of health promotion. GPs and nurses (at least prior to implementation of the Diploma in Nursing courses with their emphasis on health) were given minimal training in health promotion during their basic education. As Hope (1991:64) has said: 'Doctors are not necessarily good at delivering health promotion ... the thrust of medical education is accurate diagnosis and treatment of existing problems in a hospital setting'.

The basic preparation of nurses prior to the 1990s followed a similar pattern focused on treatment rather than health promotion and prevention. The quality of training given to nurses who said they had received training in health promotion only from their GP or only during their basic nurse training, would therefore be questionable. Health promotion and prevention are considered to be key issues regarding the nation's health (DoH, 1992). There is a need, therefore, to ensure that all health workers are adequately trained to offer the appropriate advice at all times.

The study found that practice nurses work mainly with the 18–65 year old age group and, in the main, with women. None said they worked mainly with the under fives and only two said that they worked mainly with the over 65 year old group. Historically, health visitors have worked with the under fives and district nurses with older people. These findings illustrate the fact that practice nurses are filling a gap by working with the age group that has until now been relatively neglected. With adequate training, practice nurses are well placed to offer effective preventive services to this group. This can only benefit the general health of the population. The findings of this study show that the bulk of the work carried out by practice nurses is directed towards women. More needs to be done to assist with improving the health status of men, either through extending the work of practice nurses or by establishing new services.

Conclusion

In this chapter I have featured certain findings that came out of my survey. These indicate how practice nursing is becoming established as a career option for nurses, but one for which they are still largely inadequately trained and often inappropriately employed. In my report I recommended that the contracts of employment and job descriptions of practice nurses should be reviewed and guidelines issued to practices. Particular attention should be paid to the number and grading of practice nurses needed given the characteristics of practice populations. HAs should appoint nurse advisers to support the development of the work of practice nurses. The NHS should establish a register of practice nurses and should review the cost-effectiveness of their work.

Regarding their training, there is no requirement for statutory training for practice nurses to assist them to undertake their work, as there is for other members of the PHCT such as health visitors, district nurses and GPs. Health professionals who have not had appropriate educational preparation for work in PHC may be offering the practice population a poorer quality of health care.

In particular, as the analysis in this chapter has shown, practice nurses are being asked to undertake health promotion work for which they are not adequately trained. The practice population will be disadvantaged because it is less likely that they will be given the correct health education and guidance necessary to help them improve their health status. The World Health Organisation states that: 'Individuals, families and communities should receive the best possible and most appropriate preventive, health promotive, diagnostic, therapeutic, rehabilitative and supportive care in a manner that is acceptable to them'. (WHO, 1985:118)

In reviewing the current training needs of practice nurses, I concluded my report by recommending that a structured training programme should be developed for practice nurses. This should include the allocation of funds and time, the provision of supported open, distance and practice-based learning opportunities (including the effective dissemination of information about these opportunities, see Chapter 6), and the appointment of experienced practice nurses as trainers and assessors. An individual annual performance review should be instituted to monitor the educational achievements and needs of practice nurses.

If more consultation were to take place and population needs assessed (see Chapter 15), practice nurses could play their part within the PHCT, in the development of services that meet proven needs. They could provide back-up for those members of the team who have specialist skills in areas such as child health surveillance, childhood immunisations and the over-75 assessments. Also a planned, co-ordinated approach would sanction funding to train practice nurses to develop skills and expertise in neglected areas such as PHC services for the neglected middle aged groups. All this would contribute to improved teamwork.

If the NHS is to achieve an improvement in the nation's health, it needs to ensure that the skills that the nursing profession has to offer are valued and effectively deployed. Appropriate funding should be made available to develop the skills of this rapidly expanding group of nurses so that they can play their part in raising the health status of all age groups in the population.

References

Atkin, K., Lunt, N., Parker, G. & Hirst, M. (1993) *Nurses Count: A National Census of Practice Nurses.* Social Policy Research Unit, University of York, York.

Bolden, K.J. & Takle, B.A. (1984) *Practice Nurse Handbook.* Blackwell Scientific Publications, Oxford.

Davies, G. (1993) *Report on the role and training needs of practice nurses.* TCV Project Report. TCV, Welsh Office, Cardiff.

DoH (1992) *The Health of the Nation: A Strategy for Health in England.* HMSO, London.

Hope, S. (1991) Nurses can make health promotion pay its way. *General Practitioner*, 18 October, p. 64.

Stilwell, B. & Drury, M. (1988) Description and evaluation of a course for practice nurses. *Journal of the Royal College of General Practitioners*, **38**, 203–6.

UKCC (1986) *Project 2000: A New Preparation for Practice.* UKCC, London.

World Health Organization (1985) *Targets for Health for All.* WHO Regional Office for Europe, Copenhagen.

Chapter 12

Testing Learning Methods for GPs

Helen Houston

A major aim of TCV was to enable those working in the area to participate in relevant and effective education. A new principal in general practice will have spent five or six years as an undergraduate, completed one year as a pre-registration junior hospital doctor, and have satisfactorily completed three years in vocational training: two years spent as a junior hospital doctor, one year as a trainee GP. Some will have additional experience either within hospital or community medical work. Throughout these nine (or more) years, the doctor will have received a substantial amount of education and training. All work will have been carried out under supervision, and many will have undertaken additional study and acquired postgraduate qualifications. Now, as a General Medical Practitioner, the new principal must take responsibility for his or her own continuing education and must find the time to do so. Traditionally this has been achieved by undertaking courses, attending lectures or seminars at postgraduate centres, reading, discussion with colleagues and participation in the educational activities of the Royal Colleges and other local medical societies.

The 1990 GP Contract brought considerable change to primary health care. It brought changes in the organisation of services and in workload by including, for example, health promotion and disease prevention, in addition to a continuation of all general medical services. The workload of PHC teams also increased with the expectations engendered by the introduction of Patient Charters.

Changes in the provision of education opportunities

As regards education, the intended remuneration of each GP has been reduced to create the capacity to pay the PGEA to those GPs attending a balanced spread of accredited courses. CME tutors, charged with providing the relevant educational opportunities for local GPs, were introduced. Although this role had previously been undertaken by GPs, the responsibilities of the new CME tutors were far greater and, in addition, they were expected to generate the income to fund themselves (though later this expectation disappeared). There was therefore a sudden demand from GPs for accredited education, and a call from the CME tutors for help in providing such education.

Several concerns were expressed about the nature of the new continuing medical education for GPs (Mulholland, 1990). Would the 'carrot' of the PGEA distort the voluntary nature of participation in education? Would the lectures by experts lead to less collaboration between learner and provider? Harden and Leidlaw developed a series of principles that should apply for this education to be effective: convenience, relevance, individualisation, self-assessment, interest in the material, and speculation by practitioners (Harden & Leidlaw, 1992). There is little evidence that attendance at traditional courses improves performance, and the need for a variety of educational methods allowing doctors to participate in those which suit their individual learning styles is still evident (Hayes, 1995).

Among the 370 GPs working in the TCV area, there was a high proportion of single-handed practitioners, and those who do work in group practices usually work from several surgeries in order to try to bring their services closer to the population served. This population contains large numbers of people with depression and with chronic disease, particularly respiratory disease, and this creates an extremely high workload for PHC teams. Though some of the GPs' premises are excellent, many have structural and functional problems. Often there are inadequate facilities for attached staff, who find it equally hard to work from several premises.

Although general practitioners have access to their local postgraduate centres, work pressure and the difficulties of road travel (see Chapter 1) preclude most from making a regular commitment to attend postgraduate events. Liaison with those in secondary health care is therefore proportionately harder than for most urban practices. Moreover, within the same time period, there have been considerable problems in secondary care in South Wales resulting from inadequate resources and staffing.

The educational strategy of TCV

It was decided that one way that TCV could contribute to the development of PHC was through the provision of effective and acceptable educational opportunities for GPs.

The strategy was underpinned by the belief that, to be successful, the education provided should build on and complement existing learning opportunities: if at any level it was perceived that there was competition between TCV and existing provision, then we would be deemed to have failed. To achieve this, the first steps were to develop working relationships with the CME tutors in the area and also with the GPs themselves. The following objectives were set:

- identify the educational needs of the GP;
- use a variety of educational methods covering diverse subjects;
- involve the CME tutors in its delivery;
- support the CME tutors;
- pilot the education where possible;
- evaluate all educational provision.

In addition, we would disseminate guidance about what had been found to be the successful methods.

Educational needs assessment

A variety of methods were employed to determine the educational needs of the GPs in the TCV area. An initial snapshot was provided by a series of open roadshows. As well as establishing personal contact and generating discussion, particularly with local opinion leaders, a section of the roadshows was devoted to needs assessment by questionnaire and self-assessment quizzes. At the time, the CME tutors were also undertaking their own local needs assessment and were in the process of planning educational programmes. As well as an initial snapshot picture of their educational needs, it was recognised that an ongoing assessment was needed and that this would have to be built into the programme. So, following this initial exercise, assessments followed each educational activity, both related to the particular activity and to more general needs.

The results from these various sources of information revealed that there were a wide range of topics about which general practitioners perceived they had an educational need. These covered clinical areas such as: ischaemic heart disease, child health surveillance, respiratory disease, skin problems, eye problems and the care of older people, and non-clinical topics such as: audit, business planning and practice management.

Educational methodology

The objectives of the educational methods chosen were:

- to respond to the needs revealed by the assessment;
- to be appropriate to the content;

- to be evaluated for acceptability and effectiveness; and
- to enable participation from GPs currently not attending lectures based in postgraduate centres.

Serious attention was given to the provision of a range of distance learning courses that would meet these objectives. The advantages of distance learning are: (a) participants can undertake the education at a time, place and pace to suit themselves; (b) they can repeat if necessary; and (c) there is full confidentiality for each participant's pre- and post-course performance. The disadvantages are: (a) the enormous resource implications in developing the materials and providing feedback; (b) if the courses are undertaken alone, they do nothing to reduce the isolation of GPs; and (c) there is a lack of personal contact between learner and teacher.

Distance learning courses relevant to general practice were developed on the following topics: dermatology, ophthalmology, and the management of ischaemic heart disease in older people. In addition, a course on the management of child abuse in PHC was designed for use by GPs and other team members. All included pre- and post-course assessments, written materials and either audio or video material, participation in problem solving exercises, and feedback to the participants on concluding the course.

Ophthalmology for GPs

This course is now described in detail as a case study, the findings being representative of those from the other courses. This distance learning package evolved from an audit undertaken within general practices, was developed by an ophthalmologist and a GP educationalist, was piloted, evaluated, amended and then disseminated.

Eye problems in general practice are very common. They account for 1.5% of all general practice consultations (Sheldrick *et al.*, 1993). Medical undergraduates receive some teaching in ophthalmology, but the postgraduate training period for most GPs does not include any specific experience with eye problems other than that gained during the general practice trainee year. Teaching by the GP trainer, in conjunction with available literature, is supplemented by some formal educational activities either on a half-day release course for those during training or as part of a GP's education programme.

There is some evidence that the management of eye problems in general practice could be improved. Perkins (1990) studied the outcome of patients referred to their GPs by optometrists and concluded that some referrals to ophthalmologists might be avoided if GPs received improved training in ophthalmology. Harrison *et al.* (1988) found that ophthalmic opticians were more likely than GPs to refer correctly patients with suspected glaucoma and diabetic retinopathy. Rosenthal (1992) has described the expected increase in eye problems within the population, and drawn attention to technological developments in ophthalmology. He describes the potential for more referral for surgical interventions and draws attention to the length of existing waiting lists. There are of course many other reasons for referral, and it will be a challenge for GPs to ensure appropriateness.

For CME to be both relevant and effective it is important that it includes problems that are either particularly common in general practice or are of great importance to the health of the patient. Most educationalists would support the view that GPs should be responsible for this education and involved in its provision. The optimal way to determine such education is to link its development with audit undertaken by GPs themselves (McWhinney, 1989; Irvine & Irvine, 1991).

Audit

In the first phase of this project, an audit of all eye problems presenting in thirteen general practices over a one month period was undertaken. The audit involved both general practice principals and trainees. Details of the presenting eye problem, the actual management and any specific skills used were recorded; also whether or not the doctor perceived that he/she had the necessary knowledge or skills to deal appropriately and confidently with the problem. The results were collated and discussed at meetings with the ophthalmologist and GP educationalist. One meeting was with trainees, the second was with principals. By discussing the management and the self-perceptions of necessary knowledge and skills, a consensus of agreement of the required levels was attained. The educational needs of both groups were then defined and, as the results from the two groups were so similar, further developments were the same for each.

The audit exercise determined both the content and optimal method of learning and, as a result, a package was developed using (a) videotaped material to demonstrate clinical method and physical signs, and (b) an accompanying book which concentrated on factual knowledge and some reference material. The package was designed for use either by an individual or by a small group.

The pilot

The package was piloted by twelve trainees and twenty principals in practice in South Glamorgan, and was evaluated by the following methods.

- Sustained cognitive change was measured by the application of multiple choice questions. Before receipt of the package, 30 multiple choice questions were used (MCQ_1). Two months later, participants were given 60 questions, 30 being identical to the first (MCQ_1) and the other 30 covering the same topics but with different questions (MCQ$_2$).

- The participant's feedback on the content, presentation and format of the educational material was obtained verbally and by questionnaire.
- Each participant's management intentions regarding six different clinical situations were determined before receipt of the package and two months afterwards.
- Each participant's confidence in managing five separate clinical entities was similarly measured before and two months after the package.

The pre-package MCQ$_1$ was completed by 31 doctors, the post package MCQ$_2$ by 27 doctors. From a maximum of 30, the average mark increased from 12.1 to 18.8, a significant increase in knowledge sustained over two months. The numbers were too small for more detailed analysis but the improvement appeared to be general and not confined to specific topics. There was no significant difference between the marks obtained in MCQ$_1$ and MCQ$_2$, the questions that made up the post-course assessment. No check could be made by the authors that the participants did not repeat the package immediately before completing the second MCQ but it was felt unlikely as the complete package would have to have been repeated which would have been time-consuming. If any had done so then this might have served to reinforce the education they had undertaken.

Questions about the content and presentation of the package were answered by 25 participants. All but two felt that the content of the package was just right and, while most felt the presentation was good, a minority of ten of the 25 thought the presentation was only 'average'. Additional comments included with the feedback were valuable and suggested several alterations in presentation. Most of these were incorporated during the changes made to the package before distribution in the TCV area.

The management intentions were listed for six situations. Participants were asked whether for particular conditions they would usually undertake management in general practice or refer to an ophthalmologist. For example, they were asked: Would you undertake a cover test yourself? Would you usually manage chronic glaucoma in general practice? Desired responses to these situations had previously been established at a mid-audit consensus meeting. There was a significant increase in agreement with the consensus, from the pre-package average of 4.6 times (out of six), to the post package average of 5.1 times. The confidence of GPs in managing a range of eye problems did not alter significantly, however. The package itself was changed in the light of the evaluation, and each of the original participating practices was given a package for further use.

Dissemination

Under the next phase of the project, the amended package was offered to all GPs working in the TCV area. The evaluation of this phase was based on:

- uptake and completion rates;
- sustained cognitive change as indicated by the pre- and post-MCQs, assessing change for each of the six topics included; and
- participants' management intentions regarding clinical situations were determined before and after the package.

A total of 202 GPs took up the offer (54%) and, of these, 120 (59%) completed the package and returned the post-course MCQ. This showed that there was a significant increase in correct responses for 23 of the 24 knowledge questions included in the MCQ. The questions were then grouped for each topic (Table 12.1). This shows an improvement in knowledge in all six areas. This was most marked in the area of visual problems and least in regard to ophthalmoscopy. The percentage of respondents giving correct management decisions rose significantly from 64% pre-course to 78% post-course.

Table 12.1 The percentage of respondents answering four knowledge questions correctly for each of six topics pre- and post-course

Topic	Pre-course	Post-course
Glaucoma	65.0	89.2
Squint	46.2	85.0
Visual problems	54.2	90.7
Wet/dry eye	43.5	82.2
Acute red eye	61.2	88.7
Ophthalmoscopy	56.2	77.2
Total (= 100%)	202	120

The percentage answering correctly post-course was significantly greater than pre-course for all six topics ($p < 0.01$).

Discussion

The need for continuing medical education is universal and, in order to be effective, it should build on existing knowledge and skills, should be related to perceived need, and should be available through different kinds of learning experiences. It is generally accepted that self-directed learning is one of the most effective methods of adult education. Those who take the initiative for their own learning, learn more and better than others, and they are superior at using and retaining the knowledge and skills learned. Self-directed learning is based on the requirements of participants, determined according to their particular work and situation. However this does not necessarily mean studying alone or totally unsupervised (Keinanen-Kiukaanniemi, 1992).

In this study, the initial audit undertaken by a group of GPs and their trainees, ensured that the content and presentation of this distance learning package on ophthalmology was relevant to the learners' needs as a group.

It was well received with good feedback on the relevance of the content. The uptake rate amongst the GPs in the TCV area was very good, but the completion rate was disappointing. This was despite the attraction of PGEA points, the absence of cost to the participants, and the fact that the education materials were produced locally. It is not known to what extent some of those who did not take it up may have used the package without enrolling. For example, participants were able to keep the package as a resource in their practice, and partners or colleagues may have taken advantage of this. The poor completion rate has been considered in depth (Middleton *et al.*, 1992). Research has shown that drop-out from distance learning courses is associated with many factors (Kennedy & Powell, 1976).

Eye problems are common in general practice (Sheldrick *et al.*, 1992, 1993), but GPs' confidence and their ability in dealing with them is variable (Perkins, 1990; Harrison *et al.*, 1988). During the development of this package the group discussions produced consensus statements regarding the management of many eye problems and the required knowledge and skills needed by GPs. The identified needs were then addressed by the package. The evaluation, carried out in two phases, showed an increase in knowledge measured after two months, and the later analysis showed that this increase was apparent for all the six topics included. The differences before and after the package were statistically significant, but of more relevance is the fact that the size of the change was considerable. Rosenthal (1992) has argued that GPs need to keep up-to-date with the technological advances in ophthalmology. However, there are many other reasons for referral to specialists in addition to the need to take advantage of technological advances, and these need to be recognised. This study has shown that GPs need a broad range of knowledge and skills in ophthalmology, encompassing both problems commonly seen and those where there are risks if they are not managed correctly.

It was unfortunate that we were not able to measure directly the effect of this educational package on clinical practice. The intended management for different situations was measured and showed a small but significant improvement. However, it is important that the audit cycle is completed by measuring actual clinical management and any change in that management associated with educational preparation.

These results show that this distance learning package was effective in improving both knowledge and its intended application. It addressed common and important eye problems which form a significant part of general practice workload, and which account for considerable numbers of specialist referrals. The package was successful because it related to real need, its development involved GPs and an ophthalmologist throughout, and it was made available in a format which suited the learner. Following this success in the South Wales Valleys, the package has since been made available to all GPs throughout Wales – with similar evidence of its effectiveness (Houston & Beck, 1995).

References

Harden, R.M. & Leidlaw, J.M. (1992) Effective continuing education: the CRISIS criteria. *Medical Education*, **26**, 408–22.

Harrison, R.J., Wild, J.M. & Hobley, A.J. (1988) Referral patterns to an ophthalmic out-patient clinic by general practitioners and ophthalmic opticians and the role of these professionals in screening for ocular disease. *British Medical Journal*, **297**, 1162–7.

Hayes, T.M. (1995) Continuing medical education: a personal view. *British Medical Journal*, **310**, 994–6.

Houston, H.L.A. & Beck, L. (1995) Distance learning package for eye disease. *British Journal of General Practice*, **45**, 325.

Irvine, D. & Irvine, S. (1991) (eds) The benefits of audit, or why do it? In: *Making Sense of Audit*, Chapter 2, 4–15. Radcliffe Medical Press, Oxford.

Keinanen-Kiukaanniemi, S. (1992) Teaching methods for general practice. In: *General Practitioner Education: UK and Nordic Perspectives* (eds P. Pritchard & M. Lawrence), Chapter 4, 43–7. Springer, London.

Kennedy, D. & Powell, R. (1976) Student progress and withdrawal in the Open University. *Teaching at a Distance*, **7**, 61–76.

McWhinney, I.R. (1989) *A Textbook of Family Medicine*, 359-61. Oxford University Press, Oxford.

Middleton, D., Edwards, P. & Houston, H.L.A. (1992) *I've started so I'll finish: GPs and drop-out rates from distance learning packages.* TCV Discussion Paper 12. TCV, Welsh Office, Cardiff.

Mulholland, H. (1990) Continuing Medical Education – is there a crisis? *Postgraduate Education for General Practice*, **1**(2), 69–72.

Perkins, P. (1990) Outcome of referrals by optometrists to general practitioners: an 18 month study in one practice. *British Journal of General Practice*, **40**, 59–61.

Rosenthal, A.R. (1992) The demand for ophthalmic services. *British Medical Journal*, **305**, 904–5.

Sheldrick, J.H., Vernon, S.A., Wilson, A.D. & Read, S.J. (1992) Demand incidence and episode rates of ophthalmic disease in a defined population. *British Medical Journal*, **305**, 933–6.

Sheldrick, J.H., Wilson, A.D., Vernon, S.A. & Sheldrick, C.M. (1993) Management of ophthalmic disease in general practice. *British Journal of General Practice*, **43**, 459–62.

Chapter 13

Feeling Uneasy About Research

Rachel Pritchard

This chapter discusses a number of issues concerning the roles of practitioner and researcher in PHC. It is based on a descriptive study of the 'elements of district nursing practice' conducted between 1992 and 1993. My interest in this subject stemmed from working for ten years as a district nurse, and this experience seemed to provide a firm foundation from which to conduct the research. In September 1990 I was appointed as a full-time clinical fellow with TCV and decided to undertake a project on the work of district nurses.

There were two main reasons for the study: first to increase understanding of the district nurse's role and thus to promote the more appropriate use of their skills within the primary health care team. Secondly, there is a need for nurses to voice and promote the contribution they can and do make to the nation's health (Stilwell, 1991; RCN, 1992; NHSME, 1993) and to PHC (Bryar, 1994). It is argued that this contribution is not 'recognised or valued' (RCN, 1992:1), and that there is a lack of research initiated by district nurses which might develop this understanding (Mackenzie, 1989; RCN, 1992). During the course of my study, a third reason emerged: the need to understand the process of moving from being an experienced district nurse to being a research practitioner.

Becoming uneasy

This chapter focuses on this process, and the issues that arose from the experience of carrying out qualitative research into an area that was part of my own experience, district nursing practice. The findings relating to the district nursing aspects of the project have been reported elsewhere (Pritchard, 1993). The experiences of the research process raised a combination of methodological and personal issues. These emerged while collecting data for the pilot study.

Data was collected by using a topic guide to conduct unstructured interviews, which were tape recorded. Three pilot interviews were conducted in the early part of 1992 and the main interviews conducted over the latter part of 1992.

During the pilot study I began to experience difficulties. The first indication was a feeling of 'unease', which manifested itself after the first pilot interview. During the next two interviews this feeling of 'unease' grew stronger and for a while I did not want to continue with the research study. There was a six month gap between the pilot and the main study. This was partly caused by problems in accessing the organisation and persuading district nurses to volunteer to be interviewed but, more than anything, it was due to my own lack of motivation. This time was spent immersed in the literature in a search for some possible indicators as to why I should feel this way. This chapter examines three tentative explanations:

- The approach to, and the process of, qualitative interviewing which was advocated by the selective literature was felt to be inappropriate.
- I was experiencing problems of researching an area with which I was too familiar.
- I was feeling the loss of role identity, rejection by district nursing colleagues, and role conflict.

These possible explanations will be considered in the following sections: methods issues; issues relating to the relationship between the researcher and her own culture; and personal issues.

Methods issues

In the pertinent literature on qualitative research methodology there are two very contrasting views regarding the approach of the interviewer. Some authors emphasise 'detachment' while others emphasise the value of 'rapport and participation' during the interview. The selective literature that I initially used as reference strongly advocated a neutral approach, with researchers keeping their own opinions to themselves, to prevent them influencing the participants' knowledge base and, subsequently, their replies (Brenner, 1985; Field & Morse, 1985; Chenitz, 1986; Swanson, 1986). These authors advocate the 'detached' approach and suggest that answering questions and engaging in discussion should be left to the end of the interview, and that the interview process should be conducted in a 'detached' manner.

This approach I found was totally out of character. In relating to other people I had been moulded by my past life and nursing experiences, during the course of which I had to adopt numerous roles. From these experiences a multitude of personal views and opinions have emerged. To suddenly be required to suppress these during the interviews was too much for me to cope with. Yet advocates of the detached approach advise that one should ignore all roles other than the researcher role. In this study I found it impossible to do this, because of my 'internalised style of interaction' (Wilde, 1992:239).

During the three pilot interviews, I had been trying very hard to follow this 'detached approach' and conduct the perfect textbook interview, but had failed miserably. What was causing the feeling of unease was a sense of guilt and anxiety. I felt guilty because I had not succeeded in adopting the neutral stance and keeping my opinions to myself. Anxiety compounded the feelings because it was felt that unless the study was conducted according to the book, then it would not be valid. Discussions took place at this time with colleagues in TCV as other clinical fellows, particularly some of the short-term fellows who were undertaking studies with their own populations, were experiencing similar difficulties. The outcome was a discussion paper on the subject which helped to clarify the issues at the interface between the knowledge of the practitioner and the research process (Bytheway, 1992).

Further reading of the literature showed that there was a completely contrasting view to this 'detached' approach. Benoliel (1975) suggested that the interview, which involves human beings with all their values, ideas and culture, should be seen as a process of negotiation between the researcher and the participant. Oakley (1981) and Burgess (1984) claim that it is perfectly reasonable to discuss situations and ideas with participants. The researcher should create an atmosphere conducive to open discussion and there is a need to relate to participants on their own terms (Benoliel, 1975; Taylor & Bogdan, 1984). The researcher needs to remain flexible and adapt to each role as the situation demands (Benoliel, 1975). These authors advocate the 'participatory approach' to interviewing. They consider that to refuse to relate to the participants on their own terms spoils the rapport and trust that need to be built up. The use of personal experiences in the interviews is crucial to their success (Spradley, 1979; Burgess, 1984).

Taking into consideration the arguments put forward by these two contrasting views, I decided to adopt the 'participatory approach' because these views were more in keeping with my personal values, and allowed me to be natural and relaxed. Moreover, this approach was more in keeping with the overall developmental strategy of TCV and the collaborative methods that were being used in other projects (see Chapters 7, 14 and 18).

Although the feelings of guilt passed with the decision to adopt the 'participatory approach', a level of stress and anxiety remained. The interview situation sharpened my awareness that there was a difference, whatever the approach, between having a discussion with district nurses as a colleague and as a researcher.

It has been argued that the interview creates a situation that is new and unfamiliar for the interviewees and they feel and are made to feel unequal (Cornwell, 1984). The research interview was also a situation that was new and unfamiliar to me as an interviewer and I continued to feel unequal to the district nurses. Every attempt was made to bring equality to the interview situation. The interviews were designed not as a question and answer session, but structured in such a way as to encourage the district nurses to tell their own stories through dialogue – a shared attempt to understand and describe the complexities of her own district nursing practice. I was concerned to obtain an accurate account of practice reality, not an account of the professional public image. To get the dialogue going and sustained on equal terms proved very difficult. The district nurses' replies were often very brief and superficial, with long silences, even though I tried to encourage them to elaborate, using verbal and non-verbal cues. This did not appear to work. I found myself giving examples of the kind of depth of answer that I was hoping for, filling the silences with 'comparing experiences'. This immediately had the effect of 'leading' the participant and possibly causing bias.

The relationship between the practitioner researcher and his/her practice discipline

There appear to be two main problems in conducting research in a familiar setting. These are shared professional knowledge and a familiarity with the responses given during the interviews.

Although I was not currently practising as a district nurse during the study, my professional knowledge caused a problem. I traded on my identity in the hope of getting good rapport, co-operation and more in-depth information. This caused a problem when I tried (as advocated by the literature) to clarify meanings behind certain references made by the participants during the interviews. I was confronted with verbal and non-verbal expressions of doubt as to my integrity as a district nurse. I felt that the district nurses were wondering if I was plain stupid, not a district nurse as I had claimed, or if I was testing them in some way. I felt most uncomfortable using this approach, as it felt like a game of 'let's pretend'.

Reed (1991) focused on the work of nurses on three geriatric wards in a study which she undertook while practising as a nurse herself. One of the three problems she identified was the issue of 'personal knowledge' and she experienced similar problems to myself when attempting to clarify meanings. Spradley (1979:51) reflected my experience in noting that the participants feel that 'you may be trying to test them in some way'.

'Testing them in some way' appeared to be the consensus view of the district nurses. In the current climate of change, the district nurses felt threatened about their jobs and perceived my questioning them about their work to be an attempt to de-skill and cut posts. My affiliation to a Welsh Office funded project, and to the University of Wales College of Medicine, fuelled these fears. Once I became aware of these views, I deliberately brought the issues into the open prior to the start of the interview and explained the reasoning behind 'not taking meanings for granted'. This approach helped to a certain extent to allay their fears and to win their co-operation.

In this study, I found that the district nurses' responses to my questions were very obvious and familiar. Although the responses were brief and superficial, I knew 'what else' went with the answer. Obviously, the 'what else' could not be taken for granted and, as a result, I was disappointed and bored with the interviews. I knew that there was much more to district nursing than was indicated by the replies given by these district nurses. I was concerned about writing a report that contained nothing new or nothing in-depth, and about making assumptions regarding the unspoken elements of the nurses' work.

Martin (1987), in her study of how general cultural processes affect women, carried out 165 interviews with women of varying class and ethnic origins. During the interview process and afterwards she found that she experienced similar problems. The women's replies at first seemed like common sense, and she did not experience any sense of mystery over what the women said. Their replies fitted perfectly with apparent 'reality'. For many weeks she was disappointed that the information gained at the interviews did not reveal anything other than what she already knew or could read in a textbook. Eventually she realised that these facts, although familiar, required explanation. She was surprised that it took so long to recognise this, but acknowledged how difficult it can be for someone from the same culture to unearth 'taken for granted' elements (Spradley, 1979).

In my study, the real threat to valid data collection, was the degree to which I identified with many of the district nurses' experiences, and the familiarity of their responses. This threat posed two questions:

- Did I omit to discuss the 'taken for granted' elements of district nursing practice because of its tacit nature?
- Did I project some of my own reactions and experiences, rather than listen openly to theirs?

There was not much I could do about the familiarity of the district nurses' responses. Yet, I considered that the social identity that I shared with the district nurses allowed me to understand, at an intimate level, the unspoken elements and experiences of district nurses' work – the 'insider' view (Reed & Procter, 1993: 1).

Martin (1987), through experience, was fortunate enough to realise that the familiar facts required explanation and proceeded to explain. I was not so fortunate. I realised that the work of district nurses required explaining but, through inexperience as a researcher, I was unable to untangle all the elements of district nursing practice. I was unable to present it in such a way that would be valid and readable, given the complex processes that make up district nursing practice. The physical acts of district nursing are visible to any observer. What is not visible are the thought processes and the rationale that run alongside. This brought home to me the words of Douglas (1976: 106), who stated that: 'The best sociologists have always recognised that it is not wise to study what was too close to their hearts because they could not be open to the experience'. This statement made me reflect, yet again, on the research process and to question the wisdom of my choice of topic for investigation.

Possibly, as Reed and Proctor (1995) argue, greater debate is needed about the value of the perspective that the practitioner brings to research in their area of expertise, so that this experience can be used in a way which enhances and enriches research, rather than being perceived as a barrier to achieving high research standards.

Personal issues

Kram (1988) argues that one's personal characteristics – age, gender and professional group identification – have a strong effect on the definition of the problems and the manner in which the study is carried out, as well as the quality and validity of the findings.

The age and gender of the participants did not pose any problems in this study. All the district nurses were female and close to my own age. But I felt that professional group identification was in some way obstructing the collection and objective analysis of the data. The relationship that I had with the participants was an unusual one. In my view I was a district nurse acting in a temporary capacity as a researcher. The district nurses held a different view. To them, I may have been a district nurse in the past, but the past was where it remained. I was now a person to be treated with suspicion and caution: 'Can we trust her?'. This kind of reception from people whom I viewed as colleagues left me very confused. I felt hurt, rejected and without an identity. The district nurses felt that I was no longer a district nurse, even questioning whether I had ever been one. As a result I felt very vulnerable and lacked confidence during the interviews. I experienced anxiety, self-doubt and a feeling of marginalisation from the district nurses.

Throughout the study, my anxiety levels were high because I was in unfamiliar territory and unsure of the outcome. Personal values, essential to me, were threatened and I considered that I would be unable to discharge my multiple responsibilities – to the district nurses, for whom the outcome of the findings could have positive or negative effects, to my employers and, last but not least, to myself. The increased uncertainty and the risk of failure was a very strong source of personal and professional anxiety. Some of these anxieties, I considered, could be attributed to my own problems rather than the research situation itself. Others were brought about by having to confront personal weaknesses, role conflict and the forced development of a new role identity. Even so, whatever the reasons, the anxieties were very real and had to be dealt with. Reason and Rowan (1981) and Kram (1988) suggest ways of overcoming these problems through self-awareness, friendship, research supervision and use of a research team. During this study all four strategies were utilised and they helped me come to terms with the problems.

I was very aware of the factors influencing this research study; my past life and work experiences shaped my current values and perspectives. My inexperience as a researcher, however, did not allow me to measure the extent and the effect of these factors on the study, other than to acknowledge that my experiences and 'insider view' (Reed & Procter, 1993:1) enriched my understanding of the data. Friendship and support was provided throughout the research study by colleagues in TCV. These friends enabled me to complete the study. Formal project supervision was achieved through meetings with a designated supervisor in TCV, discussions with others in TCV and through presentations at TCV seminars.

Research teams may be constituted to undertake one piece of work or to work on a variety of projects. In the case of TCV, individuals pursued their own projects within the overall framework of the whole programme (see Chapter 1). It may be argued that joint projects or team projects would have been more effective in developing individuals' research skills and helping to overcome some of the problems described here. Support, friendship and informal supervision was provided by the group who between them had considerable experience of PHC and research. Thus TCV was an information resource both to practitioners in the Valleys and also to ourselves; something which was particularly important for me.

Conclusion

This is a personal account of the events, experiences and feelings that I encountered during the period of the research study. It is by no means exhaustive. Its aim is to support and inform other practitioners carrying out research, so that they do not feel 'alone' should they be subjected to similar experiences. Conducting the research study is a learning experience, whose value can never be gained just by reading the literature. I learned to read other research studies with a better awareness, to question the views expressed in the literature and to consider alternative views. My only regret is that I was unable to do justice to describing the 'elements of district nursing practice', where good, valid research, is badly needed.

References

Benoliel, J.Q. (1975) Research related to death and the dying patient. In: *Nursing Research* (ed. P.J. Verhonick), **1**, Chapter 6, 189–227. Little-Brown, Boston.

Brenner, M. (1985) Intensive interviewing. In: *The Research Interview – Uses and Approaches* (eds M. Brenner, J. Brown and D. Canter), Chapter 7, 147–62. Academic Press, London.

Bryar, R. (1994) *Nursing Outcomes of Teamcare Valleys*, Welsh Office, Cardiff.

Burgess, R.G. (1984) *In the Field: An Introduction to Field Research.* George Allen and Unwin, London.

Bytheway, B. (1992) *The Interview in Practitioner Research.* TCV Discussion Paper 10. TCV, Welsh Office, Cardiff.

Chenitz, W.C. (1986) The informed interview. In: *From Practice to Grounded Theory: Qualitative Research in Nursing* (eds W.C. Chenitz and J.M. Swanson), Chapter 7, 79–91. Addison-Wesley, Wokingham.

Cornwell, J. (1984) *Hard-Earned Lives.* Tavistock, London.

Douglas, J.D. (1976) *Investigative Social Research*, Sage Publications, London.

Field, P.A. and Morse, J.M. (1985) *Nursing Research – The Application of Qualitative Approaches.* Chapman & Hall, London.

Kram, K.E. (1988) On the researchers' group memberships. In: *The Self in Social Inquiry* (eds D.N. Berg and K.K. Smith), Chapter 12, 247–65. Sage Publications, Newbury Park.

Mackenzie, A. (1989) *Key issues in district nursing: the district nurse within the community context.* Paper 1. District Nurses Association, London.

Martin, E. (1987) *The Woman in the Body: A Cultural Analysis of Reproduction.* Open University Press, Buckingham.

NHS Management Executive (1993) *Nursing in primary health care: New World, New Opportunities.* DoH, London.

Oakley, A. (1981) Interviewing Women: A Contradiction in Terms. In: *Doing Feminist Research* (ed. H. Roberts), Chapter 2, 30–61. Routledge and Kegan Paul, London.

Pritchard, R. (1993) *The Relationship between the Researcher and the Research Process in a Descriptive Study of District Nursing Practice.* TCV Report. TCV, Welsh Office, Cardiff.

Reason, P. and Rowan, J. (1981) *Human Inquiry: A Sourcebook of New Paradigm Research.* John Wiley, Chichester.

Reed, J. (1991) *All dressed up and nowhere to go: nursing assessment in geriatric care.* PhD thesis (unpublished). Newcastle Polytechnic, Newcastle-upon-Tyne.

Reed, J. and Procter, S. (1993) *Using professional knowledge in nursing research.* Paper presented at the RCN Research Advisory Group Conference, Glasgow.

Reed, J. and Procter, S. (eds) (1995) *Practitioner Research in Health Care: The Inside Story.* Chapman & Hall, London.

RCN (1992) *Powerhouse for Change: A Manifesto for Community Health Nursing for the 1990s.* RCN, London.

Spradley, J.P. (1979) *The Ethnographic Interview*. Holt, Rinehart and Winston, New York.

Stilwell, B. (1991) *Community nursing ... permission to practice?* Queens Nursing Institute Lecture. Department of Nursing, University of Manchester, Manchester.

Swanson, J.M. (1986) The formal qualitative interview for grounded theory. In: *From Practice to Grounded Theory: Qualitative Research in Nursing* (eds W.C. Chenitz and J.M. Swanson), Chapter 6, 66–79. Addison-Wesley, Wokingham.

Taylor, S.J. and Bogdan, R. (1984) *Introduction to Qualitative Research Methods: The Search for Meanings*, 2nd edn. John Wiley, New York.

Wilde, V. (1992) Controversial hypotheses on the relationship between researcher and informant in qualitative research. *Journal of Advanced Nursing*, **17**(2), 234–42.

Chapter 14

Tackling Ignorance About Leg Ulcers

Christine Rees

Leg ulcers affect one per cent of the adult population (Callam *et al.*, 1985). They can be extremely difficult to heal and there is a high incidence of recurrence (Dale & Gibson, 1986). The cost of leg ulcer treatments within the United Kingdom has been estimated at between £300 million and £600 million per annum (Thomas, 1990), but the cost to patients is immeasurable in terms of the discomfort, disability and depression they suffer. This affects all aspects of their lives, including work and leisure (Callam *et al.*, 1988).

Lewis and Cornwall (1989:82) have commented:

'Though leg ulcers can cause considerable discomfort and ill-health they are usually considered an unexciting and unrewarding condition to treat and therefore tend to receive scant direct medical attention. Much of the burden falls on community nursing staff whose degree of interest and expertise is infinitely variable.'

A district nursing sister working in North Gwent, I had a short-term clinical fellowship with TCV for one day each week between 1991 and 1992. The study that I undertook examined the level of knowledge and ignorance in primary health care concerning the assessment and management of patients with leg ulcers (Rees, 1993). Ultimately expert knowledge affects the quality of care that each patient with a leg ulcer receives.

I had observed ignorance regarding leg ulcers while working as a relief for other district nurses, and this was confirmed by becoming a member of an advisory panel whose aim was to produce a patient assessment form and management protocol for venous ulcers, and reviewing the literature for the purpose of this project.

The research instruments

To obtain the information required, three tools were used: a postal questionnaire, a structured interview and a medical/nursing record audit schedule.

The postal questionnaire was designed: (a) to determine how much training doctors and nurses had gained in relation to the management of leg ulcers, and (b) to identify who determined the standard of care and treatment for patients with leg ulcers in the community.

The structured interview was adapted from Phaneuf (1976) in order to determine:

- whether doctors and nurses were able to differentiate between a venous and an arterial leg ulcer (Lewis & Cornwall, 1989);
- whether topical treatments and dressings used were research based, efficacious and cost-effective (Milward, 1987; Pottle, 1987; Davies, 1988; Thomas & Tucker, 1989);
- whether bandages used in the community provided compression (Blair *et al.*, 1988; Thomas, 1990), and if doctors and nurses were able to apply them correctly;
- whether they were able to measure for and apply compression hosiery correctly;
- how they educated patients with venous ulcers.

The medical/nursing record audit schedule was also adapted from Phaneuf (1976). It was used, in conjunction with the nursing process (Snowley & Nicklin, 1987), to determine how the assessment and management of patients with leg ulcers were documented. The topics covered in the audit were:

- routine information including baseline observations, height, weight, urine, bloods, wound swabs, foot pulses, Doppler readings and lifestyle;
- communication;
- wound care and differential diagnosis;
- poor venous return/mobility;
- diet;
- social isolation.

Prior to commencing the study, scoring ranges were developed for the structured interview and record audit schedule. These were tested in a pilot study. A small sample of the types of practitioners to be included in the main study was drawn from another district in the county. This consisted of two GPs, two practice nurses and two district nursing sisters (both caseload holders). This enabled me to determine:

- whether access to the sites (practices, clinics and health centres) was easily obtained;
- if the tools provided the necessary data;
- the length of time the interview and the audit took to complete;
- how many of the total population could be included in the sample in the time available.

Minor adjustments were made to the instruments following the pilot study, but the main benefit was that it revealed the considerable amount of time that was needed to make contact with the practitioners, to arrange and conduct the interviews and to conduct the audit. For this reason it was decided to include a random sample of GPs and practice nurses, rather than the total population, in the final sample.

Problems and limitations of the methods used

The methods used for this study were expensive in terms of telephone calls, travelling and the researcher's time, but they were probably the most effective in terms of gaining access to the site and to relevant data. To assess professionals' knowledge and to audit patients' records, it was necessary to visit health centres and surgeries. Access was often difficult, especially to general practitioners and practice nurses. They were often busy and this could result in discovering after repeated telephone calls that the doctor or nurse was unwilling to participate in the study. Refusal could be for any of the following reasons: they were too busy, they did not wish to participate, they did not have patients with leg ulcers on their caseload, or 'the district nurse deals with them'.

For inclusion in the main study I identified random samples of 26 GPs and 19 practice nurses, and all 27 district nursing sisters who were caseload holders in the study area. In total, 13 (50%) of the GPs, 8 (42%) of the practice nurses and 26 (96%) of the district nursing sisters agreed to participate in the study. Some GPs had more than one surgery, and district nurses had home notes in patients' homes. Therefore, in a minority of cases, second visits had to be made to audit the patient records.

Morison (1991) suggests that some nurses may give excellent nursing care but are poor at documenting it, whereas the opposite may apply to others: documentation of the care given is of a high standard, but the care is poorly implemented. Ideally it would have been better if I had observed the care given as well as auditing the patient's records, but time and the size of the sample would not allow this.

Upon completion of the study, I used the information from the postal questionnaire, structured interview and record audit schedule to study the responses to each item and section. I compared the information within the three individual groups, and between the three professional groups.

Findings

From the literature it is evident that each patient with a leg ulcer should be holistically assessed, and that there should be documentation of: the assessment, the care planned, implementation, and the evaluation of the care given. Only then can continuity of care be assured (Cummings *et al.*, 1989; Chubby, 1990). Having achieved the above, members of the PHCT should be able to decide on appropriate care, which would be aimed at reducing patient discomfort through optimising wound healing and preventing a recurrence of the leg ulcer (Callam *et al.*, 1987; Moffatt & Stubbings, 1990). This would then result in subsequent financial gains to an already depleted NHS.

This study has revealed that leg ulcers are a problem experienced by people seen by members of all three professional groups (GPs, district and practice nurses). Overall, of the 47 participants, 11 saw the problem 'sometimes', 9 saw it 'often' and 27 (58%) always had patients with leg ulcers on their caseloads. Training already received by each professional group on this subject was minimal. The training of the majority of district nurses had been provided by manufacturers' representatives.

With the exception of differential diagnosis, a majority of GPs and practice nurses stated that it was district nurses who determined the treatment and standards of care for patients with leg ulcers. The district nursing sisters agreed with this, but they also felt that they were responsible for diagnosing the underlying cause of the leg ulcer. The lack of involvement of GPs and practice nurses in the care of people with leg ulcers was reflected in the results. All the sampled GPs and practice nurses had either a poor or unsafe overall score. In contrast, the majority of district nursing sisters (76%) had an average (that is safe) overall score on the assessment and management of patients with leg ulcers. Overall, however, the district nurses' levels of knowledge did not warrant the faith placed in them by the GPs and practice nurses (Table 14.1). The two areas where a majority of GPs, district and

Table 14.1 Overall scores on the assessment and management of leg ulcers

	GPs	District nurses	Practice nurses	Total
Excellent	0	0	0	0
Good	0	2	0	2
Average	0	20	0	20
Poor	9	4	7	20
Unsafe	4	0	1	5
Total	13	26	8	47

practice nurses scored poorly were in differential diagnosis and patient education.

Patient education

In relation to patient education, Nudds (1987:12) comments that:

'Patients need knowledge of their condition before they can understand their treatment and co-operate with the doctor and the nurse. They must be able to accept their leg ulcer and recognise their role in promoting health.'

Of the total sample, 21 (48%) of the GPs and nurses agreed that 'patients do not comply' with treatment. But patients cannot comply with treatment if no (or only minimal) information is given to them. A majority of the doctors and nurses (84%) had either poor or unsafe scores on patient education (Table 14.2).

Table 14.2   Scores in relation to patient education

	GPs	District nurses	Practice nurses	Total
Excellent	0	0	0	0
Good	0	1	0	1
Average	0	6	0	6
Poor	1	8	2	11
Unsafe	10	11	6	27
No records	2	0	0	2
Total	13	26	8	47

Wound care

The study revealed that as many as 40% of the GPs and nurses were still using cotton wool to cleanse wounds. In addition to this, 34% were using lanolin-based preparations and 11% using steroid-based preparations on the surrounding skin over a long period of time. One in three were not using bandages that provided compression to promote venous return, and one in four were not using dressings in accordance with manufacturer's instructions.

There were GPs and nurses who were uncertain whether to take a wound swab routinely or only if the wound was clinically infected, uncertain whether to immerse the leg in water, uncertain which dressing technique to use for a leg ulcer (aseptic or clinically clean), and uncertain how often compression hosiery should be renewed. All this demonstrates the need for a wound care policy to be drawn up and implemented in PHC.

Although GPs and nurses addressed issues such as routine information and social isolation slightly better, a majority (85%) had either an incomplete, poor or unsafe score when documenting care: how they assessed, planned, implemented and evaluated the care given, especially in relation to teaching the patient, setting desired outcomes and evaluating the care given (Table 14.3).

Table 14.3 Overall scores in recording their assessment and management of patients with leg ulcers

	GPs	District nurses	Practice nurses	Total
Excellent	0	0	0	0
Good	0	4	0	4
Incomplete	4	15	2	21
Poor	8	5	4	17
Unsafe	1	1	0	2
No records	0	1	2	3
Total	13	26	8	47

The attitudes of the study sample towards leg ulcers were reflected in some of the comments they made:

'Has always been a little bit of a Cinderella thing. One of the chronic sources of medical disappointment in general practice.' (GP)

'I wish there was a magic treatment for them all. There are too many dressings on the market to choose from.' (District nurse)

'It's a very grey area. No two nurses agree, let alone anyone else.' (Practice nurse)

Despite such negative comments, a majority of the participating doctors and nurses (92%) identified areas where they felt they needed further training on this topic. Their preferred methods of training were practical workshops, fieldwork, seminars or lectures.

Dissemination

In view of the fact that this project, based in Wales, confirms research in England and Scotland (Callam *et al.*, 1987; Mallett & Charles, 1989; Ertl, 1992) that there is a need for educational courses on the assessment and management of leg ulcers, I recommended in my report that courses should be provided to address the following issues:

- how to develop and evaluate a management protocol for leg ulcers in clinical practice;
- methods of differential diagnosis, through clinical examination and the use of a Doppler;
- how to develop a wound care policy;
- how to undertake comparative studies on wound care products;
- how to improve venous return by organising, for example, work-shops on compression bandaging and hosiery;
- nutrition and wound healing;
- the problems of social isolation;
- patient education.

All courses should be evaluated including observation in clinical settings both before and after the course.

Many of the studies undertaken at TCV provide baseline information about deficits and the need for service development. Such service development lies in the hands of service providers and commissioners. Part of the TCV strategy was to disseminate project findings widely to relevant organisations, providing them with information which could be used in service development plans. Copies were also sent to all the doctors and nurses who participated in the study.

Outcomes

Since completing the project I have taught in-service training courses which have included theory and the development of practical skills. I have also taught on a WNB course. Requests have been made for further sessions. I have also been approached by the independent sector to undertake training sessions. Unfortunately, despite there being great demand for the credit level English National Board course 'The Assessment and Management of Patients with Leg Ulcers', there does not appear to be any evidence of the WNB developing such a course.

There is a WNB course on 'Wound Management and Nursing Care' at diploma level, which includes some training on the assessment and management of leg ulcers. However, because of its diversity in addressing issues relating to a number of different wound types, the topic of leg ulcer management may not be covered adequately. Another limiting factor is that the course is only available for nurses, whereas my study has shown that the problem of ignorance in PHC concerning the assessment and management of patients with leg ulcers is multidisciplinary.

A *Wound Management Good Practice Guide* has been produced by the Wound Healing Research Unit, of the University of Wales College of Medicine, Cardiff. This includes protocols for the assessment and management of patients with leg ulcers (Wound Healing Research Unit, 1994). This good practice guide has the potential to improve the care of patients with leg ulcers through the provision of up-to-date information to all members of the PHCT.

Although I am now being used as a resource person by district nurses within the locality and in the surgery by the GPs and practice nurses, it does not seem that a systematic policy of providing training for the latter two groups will be implemented. For treatment potential to be maximised, the emphasis should be on multidisciplinary courses for GPs and community nurses. As this study has demonstrated, quality care at the present time is not assured within PHC for patients with a leg ulcer.

Conclusion

This study has demonstrated that patients with leg ulcers are not being holistically assessed. It highlights the need for GPs and nurses to be educated in relation to the assessment and management of leg ulcers. This should help to ensure that appropriate, cost-effective treatments that reduce patient discomfort through optimising wound healing and through preventing the recurrence of the leg ulcer, are prescribed.

The likelihood of an individual developing a leg ulcer does increase with age (Callam *et al.*, 1985). Demographic studies have shown that because of improved diet, housing and general standards of living, the number of older people in the population is rapidly increasing (Bond *et al.*, 1993). There is an increasing emphasis on the provision of community care rather than residential care. Unless a systematic approach is used for the assessment and management of patients with leg ulcers, the cost to the NHS will increase at a considerable rate but, much more importantly, patient suffering will be prolonged.

References

Blair, S.D., Wright, D.D.I., Blackhouse, M., Riddle, E. & McCollum C.N. (1988) Sustained compression and healing of chronic venous ulcers. *British Medical Journal*, **297**, 1159–61.

Bond, J., Coleman, P. & Peace, S. (1993) *Ageing in Society*. Sage Publications, London.

Callam, M.J., Ruckley, C.V., Harper, D.R. & Dale, J.J. (1985) Chronic ulceration of the leg: extent of the problem and provision of care. *British Medical Journal*, **290**, 1855–6.

Callam, M.J., Dale, J.J., Harper, D.R. & Ruckley, C.V. (1987) *Lothian and Forth Valley Leg Ulcer Study*. Buccleuch Printers, Hawick.

Callam, M.J., Harper, D.R., Dale, J.J. & Ruckley, C.V. (1988) Chronic leg ulceration: socio-economic aspects, *Scottish Medical Journal*, **33**, 358–60.

Chubby, C. (1990) Which dressing? *Journal of the Wound Care Society. Nursing Times*, **86**(15), 63–4.

Cummings, C., George, G., Hansen, J.F., Rowe, R., Shipes, E. & Watson, J.E. (1989) *How to Teach Patients*. Springhouse Corporation, Springhouse, Pennsylvania.

Dale, J.J. & Gibson, B. (1986) Leg ulcers: a disease affecting all ages. *Professional Nurse*, **1**(8), 213–6.

Davies, J. (1988) Healed at last. *Community Outlook. Nursing Times*, **84**(32), 11–12.

Ertl, P. (1992) How do you make your treatment decision? *Professional Nurse*, **7**(8), 543–52.

Lewis, J.D. & Cornwall, J.V. (1989) The assessment, management and prevention of leg ulcers. *Care of the Elderly*, **1**(2), 82–5.

Mallet, J. & Charles, H. (1989) *Survey of Clients with Leg Ulceration Treated by District Nurses in Paddington and North Kensington.* Department of Public Health, St. Mary's Hospital, London.

Milward, P. (1987) The use of hydrocolloid dressings for the treatment of leg ulcers in the community: drug tariff considerations. *Care, Science and Practice*, **5**(2), 31–4.

Moffatt, C. & Stubbings, N. (1990) The Charing Cross approach to venous ulcers. *Nursing Standard*, Special Supplement, **5**(12), 6–9.

Morison, M.J. (1991) The Stirling model of nursing. *Professional Nurse*, **6**(7), 366–70.

Nudds, L. (1987) Healing information. *Community Outlook. Nursing Times*, **83**(38), 12–14.

Phaneuf, M. (1976) *The Nursing Audit.* Appleton-Century-Crofts, New York.

Pottle, B. (1987) Trial of a dressing for non-healing ulcers. *Nursing Times*, **83**(12), 54–8.

Rees, C. (1993) *The Assessment and Management of Patients with Leg Ulcers.* TCV Report. TCV, Welsh Office, Cardiff.

Snowley, G.D. & Nicklin, P.J. (1987) *Objectives for Care.* Austen Cornish Publishers, London.

Thomas, S. & Tucker, C.A. (1989) Sorbsan in the management of leg ulcers. *Pharmaceutical Journal*, **243**, 706–9.

Thomas, S. (1990) Cost-effective management of leg ulcers. *Community Outlook. Nursing Times*, **86**(11), 21–2.

Wound Healing Research Unit (1994) *Wound Management: Good Practice Guidance.* Wound Healing Research Unit, University of Wales College of Medicine, Cardiff.

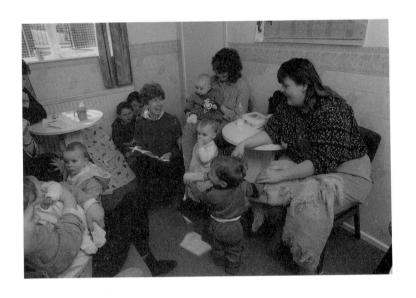

Section 4

Community Needs

All the chapters in this section are concerned directly with the needs of members of the community and of finding ways in which the PHCT could better understand and meet those needs. TCV was not directly concerned with the health of populations and did not, for example, set up projects which directly involved members of local communities. There was an assumption underlying the work of TCV that the support of practitioners in the development of PHC would lead to the better provision of services for members of the community. The projects in this section, along with those described in Chapters 19 and 22, were concerned more directly with the needs of members of the community.

Each of these projects shared an interest in reviewing the organisation of their practice and of identifying ways in which it might be made more efficient and effective, and better able to meet the needs of the local population. Their concerns ranged over the perceptions of members of the community as to the meaning of health, organisation of clinics, the most appropriate methods for patient education, patient choice, teamwork, liaison with other PHC groups, and improving access to those most in need. In their different ways they demonstrate how practitioners and PHCTs can not just undertake audit or research, but also act effectively upon the findings. It is in implementing changes prompted by research that the support of an agency such as TCV can be most effective.

In the first chapter in this section the issue of health need is explored through a study of the views of members of the practice population and the views of practice staff. The identification of local health needs should be fundamental to the work of all PHCTs, but as Chapter 15 illustrates, there may be considerable differences between lay and professional viewpoints.

Chapter 16 focuses upon the provision of patient education in an asthma clinic. In part, it endeavours to determine the most efficient use of the time of a GP and practice nurse. But it also raises interesting questions about the response of patients to the option of group education. The need for this kind of innovation to be manageable by practices with the most limited resources is emphasised.

PHC is provided primarily from health centres, surgeries and various other community facilities. The community development strategy towards raising the quality of life in deprived localities requires facilities and services to be located in them. When PHC is only available three or four miles away, the public transport system is poor and expensive, and when someone is having to cope with major demands within their own home, then a trip to the health centre is only undertaken when it seems absolutely essential. In South Wales, as in other deprived areas, there are a number of isolated housing estates where many people with major economic, social or health problems are placed by local authority housing departments. These estates often have the most minimal of community facilities. Chapter 17 describes an important project in which a local authority housing department leased an ordinary family house in such an estate, for use by a health visitor. It was a particularly challenging opportunity which required considerable diplomacy not just with the local residents but also with the management personnel of a number of different agencies.

One important aspect of the organisation of PHC is the understandings that different groups have about mutual referral practice. It is one thing to know what professional group X does and what particular skills they have, but it is another to know when and in what circumstances one should refer a patient to benefit from that group's particular service. In part referral practices build upon experience and reflect informal agreements as much as formal arrangements. From time to time, however, it is helpful if the situation is reviewed, particularly when other changes seem to have upset these understandings. Chapter 18 examines the referral of patients from GPs to CPNs. It reveals serious inconsistencies regarding the diagnosis and response to depression amongst GPs, and between GPs and CPNs.

This section identifies the need to question all aspects of PHC practice: why are particular services being provided? Are services meeting the real needs of the community? Are services being provided in the best location? Are the best methods being used to provide services? Do all members of the practice team share the same definitions? As indicated in the chapter, TCV gave these practitioners the opportunity to ask these questions and to generate answers which had a significant impact on their practice.

Chapter 15

Assessing Need

Andrea Thomas

In recent years, attention in the NHS has focused on PHC, and especially on health promotion and preventive services. These are seen to be the means of addressing many contemporary health problems. While the cost of treatment services escalates, the demand for them seems to many to be limitless. Investment in health promotion and disease prevention is expected to prove to be more cost effective. The 1990 GP Contract encouraged GPs to participate in health promotion, by introducing a sessional fee for health promotion clinics. The present bandings continue to emphasise the significance of health promotion and prevention. Obviously, for health promotion to be effective participation of members of the public is a necessity. Their motivation is more likely to be harnessed if such activities deal with issues that they deem to be imperative.

According to Bryant (1988:v), the International Conference on Primary Health Care at Alma-Ata in 1978 resulted in: 'a call for radical change in both the content and design of health services'. In defining PHC, the Declaration of Alma-Ata emphasised the importance of health promotion and disease prevention, equity of service provision, and the participation of the public in the planning and implementation of health care. It recognised the importance of understanding the needs of the population to ensure effective services, and stated that at the local level PHC relies on a health team that responds: 'to the expressed health needs of the community' (Bryant, 1988:9). The community's main health problems should be addressed, giving priority to those most in need.

PHC was seen to be the key to achieving 'Health For All' by the year 2000, and the European *Targets for Health For All* (WHO, 1985) reiterated that PHC services should respond to identified need. Target 28 stated that services should be provided: 'to meet the basic health needs of the population and give special attention to high-risk, vulnerable and underserved individuals and groups' (WHO, 1985:106). The subsequent Ottawa Charter for Health Promotion (WHO, 1986) drew attention to the necessity of adapting health promotion strategies to local needs.

Clearly the provision of effective and equitable PHC services including health promotion, requires both the assessment of health needs and the involvement of the public. These international strategies have been translated into local targets in countries throughout the world. In Wales the underlying principles of the strategy to improve the health of the population in Wales are outlined in *The Strategic Intent and Direction for the NHS in Wales* (WHPF, 1989) which places emphasis on:

- health gain
- people-centred services
- effective use of resources.

Health needs assessment plays a vital part in achieving patient-centred services. For the NHS to reach its aim of ensuring that: 'people's needs and expectations are considered when services are being planned' there must be an effective means of: 'identifying people's views on the health needs of themselves, their families and their communities' (WHPF, 1989:20).

> 'Health care needs assessment has always been necessary, but it is only in the last few years that it has assumed a central role in health service planning.... The growth in health service spending, the purchaser-provider separation, lack of evidence of effectiveness, and the uncertainty of the appropriateness of health care spending have prompted more information-intensive forms of health care needs assessment in some countries. But the UK Health Service reforms require it with some urgency.' (Stevens & Rafferty, 1994:11–12)

In recent years there has been a proliferation of studies which have involved the public in assessing health needs. For example, Dun (1989) described a community health survey carried out in Clapham, South London, and Snee (1991) described the use of a community development approach that involved local people in assessing the health needs of their community in Dallam, Cheshire. In both these studies, however, the focus was a geographically defined area where residents related to more than one general practice.

The study

With the increasing autonomy being given to PHC, typified by the growth in fundholding practices, I felt that a study exploring the views of patients and staff associated with one general practice, rather than one geographical area, could contribute to a better understanding of how a single PHCT might undertake its own health needs assessment. During the early visits that the clinical fellows made to the practices I was particularly interested in the ways in which practices identified health needs in their areas. Subsequently I wrote a discussion paper (Thomas, 1991) in which I raised a number of questions such as: Is there agreement that the public should participate in the planning and provision of health care? I concluded the paper with a request to readers for their responses to a number of questions including: Is a health needs assessment of the population served essential for the provision of PHC services?

Writing this discussion paper focused my attention on the question of how information about health needs could be gleaned from members of the practice population. I designed a study to investigate this further and I sent the discussion paper, together with tentative ideas for this project, to a number of GP practices. One of these responded to say that they would like to be involved.

The objectives of the study were:

- to undertake a perceived health needs assessment of a sample of the practice population;
- to ascertain how members of the practice PHCT perceived the health needs of their practice population;
- to make a comparison of the perceptions of the members of the practice population and the practice staff.

The study aimed to encourage public participation in order to facilitate the provision of appropriate PHC services by:

- identifying unmet health need;
- indicating the match/mismatch between lay and professional perceptions of health need;
- suggesting ways in which primary health care practitioners can 'tap the public viewpoint and encourage participation'. (Thomas, 1993:1)

I had to decide how best to elicit people's views and so I considered the various qualitative methods available. I discounted questionnaires as being too structured for my purposes and because they would not allow me to probe in depth. Abramson (1990:135) considers the use of qualitative methods to be: 'part of the process by which a practitioner of community medicine gets to know the community for which he provides care'. According to Krueger (1988:21), focus groups provide: 'information about perceptions, feelings and attitudes ... the procedure allows professionals to see reality from the client's point of view'. One advantage of this method is that it provides in depth information because the interviewer 'can follow up ideas, probe responses and investigate motives and feelings' (Bell, 1987:70). For this study, I decided that data should be collected using semi-structured interviews and focus group discussions.

My previous experience as a health visitor and health visitor lecturer, prior to becoming a full-time clinical fellow, meant that I was used to dealing with people both on a one-to-one basis and in groups. However, I felt that I needed some further preparation to enable me to undertake personal interviews and focus groups. I read up on these methods and discussed them with those experienced in their use. I observed focus groups in action and participated in a public consultation exercise which employed interview methods.

Data were collected between March and December 1992. The interviews and focus groups were taped with the participants' agreement and later transcribed. So that members of the practice population were aware of the study, a notice providing information about it was put up in the surgery waiting room.

The patients' sample

The GPs gave me access to the names, addresses, and dates of birth of their adult patients. The adult practice population was then divided into ten age-sex groups, and participants were randomly selected from within these groups. All the participants were assured of confidentiality. No-one associated with the GP practice was told which patients had been invited to participate. Seven focus groups were held and the number of participants for each group ranged up to seven. Seventeen people were interviewed in their own homes, either singly or in pairs. By undertaking this study I wanted to find out what people thought was important for their health, what they felt they needed. 'Felt need', according to Bradshaw (1972), is equal to 'want'. He argues that by itself it is an inadequate measure of 'real need'. What people feel they need can be limited by their perceptions and knowledge of available services. It can also be inflated by people asking for help without 'really needing it'. When expressing their views, participants in this study tended to use the words 'need' and 'want' synonymously.

Participants were asked if they considered themselves to be healthy. The subsequent interviews and discussions explored their views concerning:

- what does or does not contribute to health;
- what should be done either personally or by way of service provision to maintain or improve their health;
- whether they thought they should be consulted regarding the services provided for their health.

Participants were free to raise whatever issues they thought relevant.

The PHCT sample and the CHC

The GPs and the nursing and administrative staff were interviewed either singly or in pairs. The community nursing staff who work with the practice, the district nurses, the health visitors and the community midwives, were interviewed in professional groups. Community Health Councils are seen as the voice of the public and, for this reason, three members of the local community health council were also interviewed.

A qualitative research study such as this cannot represent all the views of the whole population because the number of people interviewed is too small. However, it does allow insight into the reasoning behind some people's views, and it provides a basis for further quantitative research by raising issues which can be explored with a larger number of people.

The study generated a large amount of data which has been reported elsewhere (Thomas, 1993). The following topics are discussed here: attitudes to health and lifestyles; information to the public about primary health care services and consulting the public.

Being healthy

Being healthy was viewed in the following ways:

- Not being ill enough to necessitate visiting the doctor or taking time off from work.
- Not having any physical problems. One woman said: 'I don't suffer with ill-health at all ... now and again I get panic attacks... That's not a thing that I would call unhealthy like, you know. I mean I don't suffer physically with anything'.
- Coping with a physical complaint. One man with asthma said: 'Generally yes, I think I am healthy'. He considered his asthma to be a minor problem that he was well able to control by appropriate use of medication.
- Having a healthy lifestyle.

Conversely, not being healthy was viewed in terms of physical conditions such as having respiratory and cardiac problems or an unhealthy lifestyle. Chronic diseases, namely heart disease, asthma and the industrial legacy of respiratory diseases, together with an unhealthy lifestyle, were said to be particular health problems in the area.

Looking after yourself

Views were expressed on personal responsibility for health; for example, one woman said: 'If you want to be healthy you've got to look after yourself'.

In contrast, Mr B's philosophy was summed up in the phrase: 'a mongrel will live longer than a pedigree'. He explained: 'I think if you treat your body rough you'll live till you're ninety and I honestly believe that. But if you look after yourself you die when you're fifty-five'. On this basis he was continuing to smoke and drink. He gave the example of people he used to work with: 'They've never smoked, they've never drunk and they've got cancer and died. They never chewed twist and they used to say to me "B, you'll kill yourself". But I'm still around. But all of them have gone like. So it doesn't make sense do it? It doesn't make sense'.

Davison (1989:46) has identified this as the 'Uncle Norman' syndrome: 'An aged and healthy friend, acquaintance or relative – an "Uncle Norman" – who has smoked heavily for years, eats a diet rich in cream cakes or chips and/or "drinks like a fish" '. A number of other participants put forward examples of 'Uncle Norman' figures contradicting health promotion messages.

Consulting the public

There was general agreement amongst the members of the PHCT that patients should be consulted regarding their health needs. In this way needs not previously identified can be revealed and thereby service provision improved. One receptionist remarked: 'When it comes down to it we're here for the patient and we need to know what the patient needs and expects from the practice'.

A couple of practice nurses made similar comments: 'We could always ask the patients I suppose. We set these things up and we don't actually ask the patients what they feel they need. Maybe that's a very important thing'.

'Well, the patient is what it's all about. You know at the end of the day it's whether the patient is satisfied with the service. I mean we might think it's up and running very smoothly but we don't know if it's satisfying the patients' needs and there's only one way to find out and that's to ask them.'

A district nurse agreed: 'It's good to have feedback'.

Who should be consulted?

On the whole members of the PHCT felt that both patients who attended the surgery and those who rarely made use of the service should be consulted. As one receptionist remarked: 'just because they're not sick it doesn't mean that their views don't count. I mean they're still registered with this practice.' The midwives commented that just because people were not back and forth to the surgery, that did not mean that they had healthy lifestyles. A practice nurse expressed the doubt that: 'you're not really going to get a very clear view from people who perhaps haven't been here for years'. A GP pointed out that people who attend the surgery might have different views from those who did not and to ask only the attenders would produce a biased view.

A practice nurse commented that, to be representative of patients' views, a cross-section of people should be involved. She also proposed focusing on people that the practice did not hear from, declaring: 'It's the people that don't come who are out in the community that might have health needs that we don't know about, that we need to be targeting'.

It was pointed out that people who did not attend the surgery might not know what services were available, and that they would get to know about the services through being consulted. As one receptionist stated: 'if a person doesn't visit the surgery regularly, they should still know what's going on within the surgery so that, if that service is ever needed, they should know what's available and what to expect when they get here'.

However, another viewpoint was that patients who did not attend the surgery from one year to the next did not care what services were available. Patients should make the practice aware of their needs. As one practice nurse pointed out: 'unless they come and ask for it, it's difficult to know if they need it'. On the other hand the practice should ask patients, explained one receptionist, because 'there's things people need and they, a lot of them, don't like to, sort of come forward and ask if there's something they can have'. This was especially true of the older people because: 'they are of the opinion that you shouldn't really ask', whereas: 'younger ones are getting that if they think they need something they will ask'.

Does the public want to be consulted?

Opinion was divided among members of the public as to whether or not patients should be consulted regarding their health needs and their views on what services should be provided for them. Some people felt that the doctors should decide on services. For example, Mrs U felt that the doctors knew best, and Mrs B said: 'I think it's up to the doctor myself'. Referring to the surgery, Mrs K said: 'they've done a pretty good job on their own without consulting anybody really', and Mr G said: 'if you've got good doctors like we got, I'd leave it in their hands, I would'. One older participant commented: 'As far as I'm concerned, I'm happy ... anything I've ever wanted I've had as far as my health is concerned'.

There were a few members of the practice population who expressed concern about the management of services and the involvement of the public. Mrs T thought that people should be consulted but that available resources had to be taken into account. She commented: 'you can't say, "Oh they ought to do this and they ought to do that." If the money's not there, they can't'.

Referring to GP funding and the prioritising of services, Mr D said: 'There should be a patient type involvement. What I'm afraid of is that doctors will become accountants where they will be watching the pennies rather than watching the patients'. Mr D suggested the setting up of a forum, which would include:

'... responsible people of the public who are patients ... To set up the priorities, because I feel that if it is left to the medical profession alone then cost is bound to play an important part. If it was left to, if you like patients alone, you're gonna get sentimentality creeping in. So you've gotta find the right mix to combine the two, cost-effectiveness and the, if you like, the caring to the person who needs it.'

Mr E also raised the issue of who would participate. He asked: 'Who will decide who joins? ... do you sort of draw the names out of a hat? Would they be invited and only a few turn up?' Mr D pointed out that trying to decide which patients would join was: 'going into a mine-field'.

Conclusion

The public needs information, if they are to make informed choices and access appropriate health care services. Although this GP practice published a booklet, few of those interviewed were aware of it. The onus was on those who did not regularly attend the surgery to make enquiries regarding any services they might need. As one man stated: 'unless you actually go to the surgery and read the posters, there's nothing'. Alternatively, they would possibly hear about services by word of mouth. Not everyone was happy with this state of affairs. One woman said 'I mean, it's awful to think that you've got to be ill to find out about things'.

One important lesson I learnt while undertaking this project was that obtaining the views of the public is extremely difficult. As health care professionals we may decide to consult the public but are the public able and willing to express their views? I discovered that, contrary to my expectations, many members of the public choose not to partici-pate. In discussion with colleagues in PHCTs in the area, at TCV and with others familiar with South Wales, suggested explanations for this were that the population is satisfied with services, is apathetic, lacks confidence, fears retribution, or is disillusioned with public consul-tation.

If, as health professionals, we believe that comprehensive health needs assessment should incorporate the views of the public, then these issues have to be addressed. Public participation must not become a token exercise. If we expect people to voice their needs, then we in turn should be prepared to acknowledge and respond to their views.

References

Abramson, J. (1990) *Survey Methods in Community Medicine*, 4th edn. Churchill Livingstone, Edinburgh.

Bell, J. (1987) *Doing Your Research Project*. Open University Press, Milton Keynes.

Bradshaw, J. (1972) A taxonomy of social need. In: *Problems and Progress in Medical Care. Essays on Current Research* (ed. G. Mclachlan), Chapter 3, 69–82. Oxford University Press, Oxford.

Bryant, J. (1988) *From Alma-Ata to the Year 2000. Reflections at the Midpoint*. WHO, Geneva.

Davison, C. (1989) Eggs and the sceptical eater. *New Scientist*, **121**(1655), 45–9.

Dun, R. (1989) *Pictures of Health?* A report of a community survey carried out in Clapham, South London. West Lambeth Health Authority Community Unit, London.

Krueger, R.A. (1988) *Focus Groups. A Practical Guide for Applied Research*. Sage Publications, London.

Snee, K. (1991) *Dallam on Health*. Report. Dallam on Health, Community House, Warrington.

Stevens, A. & Rafferty, J. (1994) Introduction. In: *Health Care Needs Assessment: The Epidemiologically Based Needs Assessment Reviews* (eds A. Stevens & J. Rafferty), Chapter 1, 11–30. Radcliffe Medical Press, Oxford.

Thomas, A. (1991) *Is Health Needs Assessment in Primary Health Care Necessary?* TCV Discussion Paper 4. TCV, Welsh Office, Cardiff.

Thomas, A. (1993) *'That's what we're there for ... the patients'. A Qualitative Study of Perceived Health Need*. TCV Project Report. TCV, Welsh Office, Cardiff.

WHPF (1989) *Strategic Intent and Direction for the NHS in Wales*. Welsh Health Planning Forum, Welsh Office, Cardiff.

World Health Organization (1985) *Targets for Health For All*. WHO Regional Office for Europe, Copenhagen.

World Health Organization (1986) *Ottawa Charter for Health Promotion*. An International Conference on Health Promotion, November 17–21. WHO, Copenhagen.

Chapter 16

Educating Asthma Patients

Ajay Thapar

The importance of patient education in asthma is now well established and there is a substantial amount of published research work on the subject. The ideal method of patient education about asthma, however, has still not been identified. In this chapter I first present the findings of my research project, which was carried out in a PHC setting, and which compared the effectiveness of two different methods of patient education. I then detail some of the strategies used to educate asthmatic patients and highlight the information that may be appropriate for patients with asthma to help them manage their illness. Finally I summarise the advantages and disadvantages of using different patient education methods.

Background

In November 1989 I joined a single-handed practice in Aberbargoed in the Rhymney Valley as the second partner. This is a typical small Valleys town, a close-knit community about 25 miles north of Cardiff. There was a large colliery nearby which had recently shut down leading to considerable job losses among the adult male community. Many of the remaining jobs in the area are based in factories resulting in a high proportion of the employed population being female. In terms of disease, chronic bronchitis and ischaemic heart disease seemed particularly common.

I was interested in patient education and tried to teach patients about their illnesses at every opportunity. It soon became apparent to me, however, that this was often difficult during the consultation especially for chronic illnesses. Time is an important limiting factor, especially as the patient is often attending because of an acute illness which itself requires management and explanation. Giving booklets about the illness did not seem adequate in itself, because it was often the case that the books had not been opened by the next consultation or the messages had not been understood.

The establishment of an asthma clinic in our practice with the implementation of the 1990 GP Contract seemed to provide a better opportunity to educate patients about their illness. However, we were uncertain as to the best method to carry this out. Educating each patient individually when they attended the clinic seemed very time-consuming and could become very repetitive. Looking through the patient education literature it seemed that educating patients in small groups was a viable alternative. This method had been used with some success in Europe for chronic illnesses such as hypertension, and had also been used by some patient education programmes in America (Ringsberg *et al.*, 1990; Wilson *et al.*, 1993). It also seemed an economic use of time, but would it be effective?

Soon after joining the practice I attended the Welsh Audit Course being run by TCV in conjunction with the Department of Postgraduate Studies for Medical and Dental Education, University of Wales College of Medicine. As part of this I organised an audit of asthmatic patients registered with the practice. Following completion of this, I decided to apply to be a clinical fellow with TCV in order to have the time to carry out a study which would compare the effectiveness of educating asthmatic patients in small groups with individual education. My application was successful.

The study

The study was carried out on all clinic attenders over a five month period with alternate clinics being designated for either group education or individual education (Thapar, 1993; 1994). Both the doctor and practice nurse were involved in the group educational sessions. One follow-up visit for each educational session was carried out. To keep the study simple, we used patient knowledge as our principal outcome measure, but we also looked at self-rated morbidity and assessed patient satisfaction.

A new comprehensive patient education booklet, *Confidence with Asthma*, had just been produced by the National Asthma Campaign (Partridge, 1990). We not only used it as a basis for the educational sessions but also derived the knowledge questions for our questionnaire from this booklet. We piloted the knowledge questionnaire formally at two asthma outpatient clinics. Questionnaires were completed both just before the first educational session and one month after the second session.

Results

A total of 68 patients participated in the study, with 34 patients being educated in small groups and 34 patients educated individually. Individual education sessions lasted an average of 20 minutes each. Group sessions took on average 35 minutes and involved an average of five patients.

Overall, knowledge scores improved in both group and in individually educated patients after the educational sessions. There were no significant differences between the improvements in knowledge score for the two types of intervention. Patients also felt more confident in managing their asthma after the sessions and there were improvements in self-rated wheeziness. Most patients found the sessions helpful, felt they learned a lot, and did not find the sessions stressful. Interestingly, 60% expressed a preference for small group education.

Overall the total time spent on individual education sessions was 11.5 hours and that on group education sessions 3.5 hours.

Discussion

This study shows that educating patients in small groups in a PHC setting is as effective as individual education in improving knowledge of asthma. Small groups seemed popular with patients and took less than a third of the time needed for individual education. These are important considerations in achieving effectiveness and efficiency, as well as in taking account of what the patient wants.

Another advantage of using a small group is that the information given to the patient is more likely to be consistent. The groups were run by the doctor and the practice nurse working together rather than separately with individual patients and this led to a shared understanding of what advice and information patients needed.

We found that using both a doctor and nurse with groups of patients facilitated teamwork. Most activities in PHC are engaged in by a single member of the PHCT, and effective teamwork is often equated with delegation and communication exchange rather than with undertaking activities jointly. Doing things together seemed to strengthen our team. In view of the problems that have been highlighted in a review of teamwork in present day primary health care (Jones & Pearson, 1994), this is an outcome of some significance.

The experience of joining a group

Having a chronic illness can be an isolating event for the patient. Inviting patients to join a small group for educational sessions created an opportunity for them to make contact with fellow sufferers which were often maintained out of surgery. Other researchers have argued that people with asthma have much to gain from the support of other sufferers (Bytheway & Furth, 1996). This kind of peer support may have been instrumental in encouraging Jane, a patient who attended the group sessions, to comply with her treatment. Her case casts some light on the value of the group sessions.

Jane was a 16-year-old girl who had just left school and started work in a local factory. She was the only child of a local tradesman and an office worker. The household also included her grandmother who suffered with moderately severe asthma. Fairly frequent home visits from the GP were requested for the grandmother's chest complaint which she generally ascribed to an infection. I was called to see Jane one afternoon when she was noted to be breathless. Clinical assessment showed that she was having a severe asthma attack and had a peak expiratory flow rate of 220 litres per minute (which was less than half of what it should have been, given her age and height). She revealed she had had several milder bouts over the previous two years. I admitted her to hospital after explaining that this was an asthma attack. The family found this hard to believe. She was discharged a few days later on a Ventolin and Pulmicort inhaler. She was persuaded to attend our practice asthma clinic where her asthma control was often noted to be poor. The reason for this was not immediately obvious. It was only when the practice nurse (who lived near them) discovered she did not often use her Pulmicort (despite initial protestations to the contrary), that the reason for poor control became clear. Despite detailed explanations and reassurances from us, she remained adamant she was not going to use this inhaler more than once a week because it was a steroid and because she was worried about side effects.

We then began our study of patient education in asthma and she agreed to take part. She was part of the sample that was educated in a small group. She attended both group sessions with four others of varying ages and asthma histories. She was fairly quiet and did not actively participate much in the group. We were considerably surprised that, at the end of the study, she not only stated that she had found the information very helpful but she also subsequently used her Pulmicort as prescribed and her asthma control greatly improved.

This history suggests that an association with other asthma sufferers, if only for just two clinic sessions, can have a major impact on behaviour and compliance.

Educating patients

Guidance for achieving effective group work often creates a feeling that it is complicated and needs special expertise. In this project, neither doctor nor nurse had any special expertise in running groups. Although problems with certain individuals did arise, we found they could be adequately addressed without recourse to special techniques.

We found a group of four to six the most suitable for facilitating discussion and encouraging all to participate. A basic principle behind the study was that the intervention should be on a scale that could be organised in any ordinary general practice.

It has often been stated that, in managing a chronic illness, a partnership should be established between the doctor and the patient (Tuckett *et al.*, 1985). To facilitate this partnership there needs to be a sharing of information. Patients are experts on how symptoms are experienced and on the implications of the illness for the way they organise their lives. The doctor is an expert on scientific aspects of the disease, such as its aetiology, pathology, epidemiology, natural history and prognosis, and on treatment and its side effects. The transfer of information between a doctor and a patient has to be appropriate and manageable. People have different levels of knowledge, different abilities and different needs. Information transfer which does not take account of this will be less effective.

However, simply giving information is not enough, as was demonstrated by our experience of treating Jane. Patient attitudes and beliefs, and the context in which the illness occurs, are also crucial to the reactions of patients to a chronic illness. Giving information is therefore a two-way process; only by understanding what an illness means to the patient and directly addressing this, is the information that the doctor or the nurse gives likely to be effective. Otherwise the patient might consider what is offered irrelevant, or even unacceptable if it directly clashes with their belief system. In the latter case it may only be accepted if their beliefs are specifically addressed and a plausible explanation given to the patient.

It may seem to follow from this argument that information has to be negotiated on a one-to-one basis and that a group setting would therefore be inappropriate. That this is not necessarily the case became increasingly clear during our study. Patients in the group setting were more likely to signal disagreement with the information given and to express their own beliefs than were patients seen on a one-to-one basis. Whether this was because they felt empowered by the peer group or whether it occurred simply by chance, is not clear. The study has not proved that one method is superior to another, simply that the power of different techniques to elicit and convey information may not be as clear-cut as is sometimes assumed.

Giving relevant information to patients which they can assimilate is important because it also allows them to make informed decisions. Patient compliance with asthma medication has often been estimated at about 50% (Levy & Hilton, 1989), and studies have suggested that non-compliance is more often an active decision by patients and not just simple forgetfulness (Morris & Schultz, 1993). Jane's history illustrates this aspect of non-compliance. The benefits of advances in drug therapy will be negated if the patient does not comply.

Presenting information

In presenting information about asthma we first used strategies to improve the communication of medical information (Ley, 1976). More specifically we tried to:

- use short words and short sentences;
- arrange information into clear categories;
- repeat advice;
- give specific advice rather than general advice.

In addition we identified commonly held erroneous beliefs and dealt specifically with these. For example, we would say: 'Some people say inhalers are addictive. They are wrong. Research shows that ...'. Similarly we tried to make information more personally relevant: 'Who uses brown inhalers? ... These work by ...' We facilitated discussion by posing specific questions at the end of each section. Using these techniques, information on the following topics was provided:

- pathogenesis and symptoms (e.g. 'asthma equals tight tubes plus sticky phlegm plus swollen tubes, leading to tight chest and lots of phlegm');
- causes and triggers (e.g. allergens such as house dust mite, genetic factors);
- medication types (e.g. preventers, relievers, side effects);
- correct inhaler use (concepts rather than techniques – techniques were taught separately);
- self-management behaviours (e.g. what to do in specific circumstances);
- other essential information (e.g. risks of beta blockers).

Advantages and disadvantages of individual education

Through this study I have learnt that one-to-one and group education each have advantages and disadvantages. The advantages of one-to-one education are:

- it can be tailored for the individual patient;
- it is a familiar setting for health service encounters;
- it can be opportunistic;
- it provides confidentiality – patient may feel more free to ask questions;
- there is some evidence that it improves knowledge and morbidity (Crosby *et al.*, 1989; Wilson *et al.*, 1993).

The disadvantages of one-to-one education are:

- it is time-consuming;
- it can be repetitive in a clinic setting;
- patients may be anxious in a one-to-one setting;

- patients may forget a lot of the information;
- patients may find it difficult to state their own beliefs if they disagree with the information given.

Advantages and disadvantages of group education

Education in small groups has a number of advantages which make it an attractive option in the PHC setting:

- it is time efficient;
- it encourages teamwork;
- it increases the consistency of the information offered to patients;
- it is popular with patients;
- there is evidence that it increases knowledge (Ringsberg *et al.*, 1990);
- there is more evidence that it decreases morbidity than exists for other methods of patient education (Avery *et al.*, 1972; Lewis *et al.*, 1984; Clark *et al.*, 1986; Ringsberg *et al.*, 1990; Mulhauser *et al.*, 1991);
- there is evidence that it is more effective than individual counselling (Wilson *et al.*, 1993).

There are the following disadvantages, however, to group education:

- it needs organisation and cannot be provided opportunistically;
- it is an unfamiliar setting for health care encounters and initially may be threatening for staff and/or patients;
- it needs group work skills; for example, there may be problems with dominant individuals or non-participating individuals;
- it may be difficult to tailor information to individual needs;
- improved morbidity may require very intensive interventions not possible in group settings.

Conclusion

In this study we set out to compare the effectiveness of two different methods of providing education for patients with asthma, in a PHC setting. Educating asthmatic patients in small groups has been shown to be an effective method of increasing knowledge of asthma. It also has several other important advantages for the PHC team. It is an efficient use of time. It encourages teamwork. It ensures consistency in the information given to patients. It is popular with patients.

References

Avery, C.H., Green, L.W. & Krieder, S. (1972) *Reducing emergency room visits of asthmatics: an experiment in health education.* Presented as testimony at hearings of the President's Committee on Health Education, Pittsburgh.

Bytheway, B. & Furth, A. (1996) Asthma. In: *Experiencing and Explaining Disease* (eds B. Davey and C. Seale), Chapter 5, 81–112. Open University Press, Buckingham.

Clark, N.M., Feldman, C.H., Evans, D., Levison, M.J., Wasilewski, Y. & Mellins, R.B. (1986) The impact of health education on frequency and cost of health care use by low income children with asthma. *Journal of Allergy and Clinical Immunology*, **78**, 108–15.

Crosby, F.R.G., Whyte, E., Ogston, S. & Clark, R.A. (1989) Improving asthma control in general practice. *Thorax*, **44**, 344.

Jones, K. & Pearson, P. (1994) The primary health care non-team? *British Medical Journal*, **309**, 1387–8.

Levy, M. & Hilton, S. (1989) *Asthma in Practice*. Royal College of General Practitioners, Exeter.

Lewis, C.E., Rachelefsky, G.S., Lewis, M.A., de la Sota, A. & Kaplan, M. (1984) A randomised trial of A.C.T. (asthma care training) for kids. *Pediatrics*, **74**(4), 478–86.

Ley, P. (1976) *Communications in Medicine*. Oxford University Press, for the Nuffield Provincial Hospitals Trust, London.

Morris, L.S. & Schulz, R.M. (1993) Medication compliance: the patient's perspective. *Clinical Therapeutics*, **15**(3), 593–606.

Mulhauser, I., Richter, B., Kraut, D., Weske, G.. Worth, H. & Berger, M. (1991) Evaluation of a structured treatment and teaching programme on asthma. *Journal of Internal Medicine*, **230**, 157–64.

Partridge, M. (1990) *Confidence with Asthma*. National Asthma Campaign, London.

Ringsberg, K.C., Wiklund, I. & Wilhelmsen, L. (1990) Education of adult patients at an 'asthma school': effects on quality of life, knowledge and need for nursing. *European Respiratory Journal*, **3**, 33–7.

Thapar, A. (1993) *Patient education in asthma: a comparison between small group education and individual counselling*. TCV Project Report. TCV, Welsh Office, Cardiff.

Thapar, A. (1994) Educating asthmatic patients in primary care: a pilot study of small group education. *Family Practice*, **11**, 39–43.

Tuckett, D., Boulton, M., Olson, C. & Williams, A. (1985) *Meetings Between Experts: An Approach to Sharing Ideas in Medical Consultations*. Tavistock, London.

Wilson, S.R., Scamagas, P., German, D.F., Hughes, G.W., Lulla, S., Coss, S., Chardon, L., Thomas, R.G., Starr-Schneidkraut, N., Stancavage, F.B. & Arsham, G.M. (1993) A controlled trial of two forms of self-management education for adults with asthma. *American Journal of Medicine*, **94**, 564–76.

Chapter 17

Housing Primary Health Care in the Community

Lyn Fisk

The past ten years have seen a radical shift in emphasis in health care provision and in health visiting practice. The move has been toward a more consumer or client-led approach to health. Health visitors have been encouraged to examine new ways of addressing the health needs of communities and groups (Goodwin, 1988). This swing away from the individualistic approach towards the model of community-oriented health care has, in part, resulted from international pressure. In particular, the 1978 World Health Organisation Conference on Primary Health Care challenged health workers to work in partnership with individuals and groups, to enable them to define their own health needs and to encourage self reliance (WHO, 1978).

The aim of a community-oriented approach is to enable people to increase control over, and to improve, their health. Community-based work in this context does not focus on problems, it aims to promote skills, knowledge and confidence. The health worker becomes more of a facilitator, whose role is to validate, encourage and empower people to define and meet their own health needs (WHO, 1991). It has long been established that primary health care workers, working in groups in a participatory way and drawing upon experiential learning, are a powerful tool for change (Billingham, 1989).

The Community Health House

Health visitors have in the past focused largely on work with individuals and families. More recently, they have been exploring different ways of working with groups and communities. The project that I undertook aimed to meet the wider health, social and personal needs of women living on an estate, through the provision of a drop-in centre. The project sought to test the effectiveness of a community development approach to health promotion with families (Fisk, 1992). It had the following objectives:

- to engage the community in discussion and planning with regard to issues with a bearing on health;
- to provide a place that would serve as a centre for health promotion activities;
- to enlist the support of various other agencies and professional workers;
- to establish a wide range of health promotion activities on a group basis;
- to evaluate the approach and develop it according to the results of the evaluation.

To compound the poor environment, the estate has many recognisable elements of poverty and disadvantage, including low average household income, a high proportion of single parents, weak social support systems, a high rate of social difficulties and few shopping, leisure or communal facilities. These factors tend to produce a sense of isolation and a feeling that change is difficult to achieve. People living there feel they have little control over their lives.

The estate is adjacent to a village community high on the edge of a valley. The area consists largely of council properties. Most families housed on the estate were placed there because they needed emergency accommodation; they were not there by choice. Among the residents there is little sense of commitment to the community. In October 1990 Ogwr Health Unit was granted the lease of a house on the estate for two years.

Throughout the year prior to the opening of the House, a small group of women from the estate worked hard to form a committee. It later took on the task of fundraising for equipment and of planning how the House could be used. It was hoped that the committee would eventually take on full ownership of the project. This committee drew up a constitution and became known formally as the Families Association. The committee met regularly on a monthly basis and eventually obtained charitable status.

It was recognised that, if mothers were to have a break from their children to be able to take part in any activities, a creche was essential. The Families Association successfully obtained one year's funding for a nursery nurse from the Opportunity for Volunteering Scheme, and a further grant was received from the BBC Children in Need Appeal.

A series of activities were identified through discussion with the women using the House. Those that were instigated included:

- shared shopping for the preparation of a daily lunch;
- outside trips such as swimming;
- courses provided by various health professionals on topics such as: first aid, talking about feelings, ante and postnatal care, children's illnesses, nutrition, cooking, hobbies and crafts.

Social activities included strawberry picking, a barbecue, and outings, for example to a local animal centre, with the children. Jumble sales and running a handicraft stall acted as social events as well as fund-raising ventures.

The evaluation

As the above description shows, activities were initiated in the house in relation to the first four of the five objectives set for the project. The fifth, the evaluation of the approach, was more difficult to achieve. To develop the House I had been released for two-and-a-half days per week from my general caseload, some of which a colleague had taken on. I had no time to develop tools to evaluate the initiative. With the support of my manager I applied and was appointed to TCV as a short-term half-time clinical fellow for six months. My salary costs were paid by TCV and a bank health visitor appointed to my caseload while I combined work on the evaluation with work in the House.

Following many discussions, it was decided that the central purpose of the project would be to devise an assessment procedure which could be used with women before they attended the House and then again after a period of attendance. Clearly, a considerable range of process and outcome factors could have been evaluated. I decided to focus on the development of an assessment procedure that could be used as part of ongoing health visiting work with families attending the House.

The aims of the assessment procedure were to:

- determine the residents' beliefs and attitudes about their general health;
- determine the extent of their social contacts and their perception of social support;
- assess their level of self-esteem using the Battle Culture Free Self Esteem Inventory (Battle, 1988);
- formulate plans and strategies for intervention – in particular activities that were being offered in the House;
- gather baseline information with a view to repeating the assessment at a later date in order to evaluate the effects of taking part in activities at the House.

The procedure consisted of a semi-structured interview and the Battle Inventory. The interview comprised questions grouped in five sections:

- family structure and background;

- general attitudes and beliefs about health;
- social support;
- attitudes to parenting;
- attitudes to, and experience of, the Community Health House.

After the tools had been piloted, a purposive sample of 23 women was drawn from my caseload to participate in the main study. These were women who were not using the House but who, I considered, might benefit from attending. They each had at least two of the following features: single parent; isolated mother/family; child under five who might benefit from purposeful play; new to the area.

Notes were taken during the interviews which were also tape recorded with the women's permission. The following discussion is based on some of the results of the assessment procedure and my experience of working in the House.

The definition of health

Central to the whole project is the concept of health, how it is defined and what factors are perceived to affect it. Table 17.1 displays the frequency with which factors were selected by the women as having an adverse effect on health, and Table 17.2 the factors selected as promoting good health. It should be noted that lack of money, crime and violence feature prominently in Table 17.1. Behavioural factors such as

Table 17.1 The factors which were selected as having a negative effect on health (Fisk, 1992:45)

Factor	%
Crime and vandalism	70
Not enough money	65
State of the area	61
Stress and worry	61
Smoking	52
Lack of shops	48
Few facilities for the under-fives	39
State of your home	39
No paid work	30
Poor health service	30
What happened to you as a child	30
Noise	30
No leisure facilities	26
Alcohol	26
Pollution	26
Total (= 100%)	23

Table 17.2   The factors which were selected as promoting good health (Fisk, 1992:44)

	%
Good friends and neighbours	83
State of your home	61
Family support	52
Enough money	43
Good health facilities	43
Your diet	43
How you were brought up	39
Transport	39
Good sexual relationships	35
Facilities for the under-fives	35
The area you live in	30
Taking exercise	26
Total (= 100%)	23

smoking and alcohol are comparatively less important. The state of the area, stress and worry are also key factors.

Table 17.2 shows that the women considered factors concerned with emotional health and relationships to be the most important for well-being. These women, therefore, defined health as rooted in social and economic factors rather than personal behaviour and lifestyle.

These findings are in line with recent research studies that show that reference to socio-economic and environmental factors are more frequently associated with people in working class groups and may well reflect their experience of adverse living conditions (Graham, 1984; Calnan, 1986; Coulter, 1987; Farrant & Russell, 1986; Davies, 1995). In the Milton Keynes Felt Needs project lack of money was perceived as having a detrimental affect on health (Liddiard, 1988). This difference in the definition of health between the public and health professionals has been found in another TCV study (see Chapter 15). Traditionally health services and health professionals have been concerned with the provision of curative and preventative services rather than with seeking to influence the wider social and economic determinants of health. Changes in the organisation of the NHS in the 1900s may have reinforced the focused approach of health trusts. However, there is evidence that policy makers are being encouraged to take a wider view of the determinants of health and to be more active in influencing the social conditions which affect the health of communities (Benzeval *et al.*, 1995).

That the public has a wide definition of health is a very positive attribute in any area where community development activities are being considered. The health visitor who has to mediate between the two views held by the community and the health trust, however, has certain difficulties. Women living in a poor estate know that an afternoon spent out in the fresh air picking strawberries will do more for their health than a home visit from the health visitor. But how can a manager justify investment in such an outing? How will it contribute to health gain targets – the questions discussed in Chapter 9?

The users of the House

The House itself was initially viewed with suspicion by the local community. Members of the Families Association were aware of the conditions of the lease of the House and of the financial support given by the Health Unit to the project. Some residents may have felt that the House – and therefore the project – was owned by the health unit or the council. However, by working flexible hours, I was able to become involved in many activities and, with this closer involvement, a better partnership was achieved between myself and local people.

An unexpected problem that occurred was that the women who were involved early in the project became very possessive of the House, and this tended to deter other women from using it. Those working in PHC are always concerned about people who do not use a particular service that could be of benefit to them. Along with other professionals, I tried to support the users in developing skills themselves. Some attempt was made at encouraging the Newpin befriending system (Pound *et al.*, 1985). This, however, would have required more skilled training for myself and for some of the mothers.

While the presence of the core group may have deterred some from using the House, low self-esteem among women on the estate might have been another factor limiting their participation. The Inventory was used as part of the assessment procedure to measure the self-esteem of women who were not using the House but who, in my opinion, could benefit. Over half of the 23 women interviewed had low or very low personal self-esteem scores. Eight had very low scores indicating a poor sense of self-worth.

In the absence of good quality support from family or friends, women with low self-esteem find it difficult to motivate themselves to meet others even though they may be in need of support. Women living in poverty have so many problems they tend to be unwilling to make friends and thereby risk taking on more problems – they recognise that friendship requires reciprocity.

The interview schedule used in the project showed that these women, despite having few friends, did have support from their families. Interviewees were asked how many times they had had contact with their family over the two weeks prior to the interview. For the majority there was contact occurring on a daily basis either by visiting, telephoning or having family to visit. Contact with friends was considerably less. Four respondents had no contact with friends and six said they had little contact.

How one perceives support is a key concept in enhancing self-esteem and a feeling of 'self worth' (Parry, 1988). A third of the interviewees were well supported. They felt that they belonged to a family they could rely on, who accepted and loved them as they were. However, three said there was no one they felt they could rely on, and another ten thought there was no such person in the local community. These were the women who potentially stood to benefit most from the Health House.

The multidisciplinary team

From the outset I realised a multidisciplinary team of people would be essential to provide support and activities in the House. Numerous statutory and voluntary bodies were approached. Those that provided on-going support throughout the two years included a community development worker, community education tutors, psychiatric nurse therapist and occupational therapist. Some individuals approached were supportive but unable to offer their time, including the local GP. Others, including Social Services and Womens Aid, participated initially but found the numbers attending their sessions did not warrant the time spent in the House. Those most involved worked within different organisations, each with particular aims and objectives and constraints. For example, the two adult education tutors were enthusiastic about working with the women, but funds had to be raised for them to undertake this work. Women attending the House organised numerous events to raise these funds.

As a team we found we were having to resolve many financial and other management problems to maintain our work at the House. We felt that these should have been dealt with by managers within our respective organisations. Further, while we met on a regular basis with a manager from the health community authority unit, we felt that the project required a steering committee with management expertise, drawn from all the organisations involved.

Conclusion

In deprived estates where there is a high proportion of families with difficulties, there exists a need for well-organised support from a variety of sources. At present there is a tendency for social work to be fully occupied with personal crises and for GPs to focus narrowly on health problems. Health visitors alone cannot provide the preventive care that is needed.

There is a clear need for health visitors to re-orient their approach to practice and to acknowledge the valuable resources that exist within the local community (Bryar & Fisk, 1994). They should draw upon and develop the expertise that residents acquire through force of circumstance. My experiences of working in the community health house suggest that health visitors working with the aim of community development should be prepared to set aside their status as 'experts'; to be flexible, honest and willing to share their knowledge and experience; and to be well informed about where other relevant information and expertise can be found.

This project illustrates some of the issues that need to be addressed if health visiting is to adopt this more participatory approach to work at the community level. Health visitors need to develop new skills and they need support in using these skills. Managers and health visitors need to explore new ways of recording outcomes of health visiting practice, moving away from counting contacts to measuring the quality of these contacts (see Chapter 9).

Health visiting has developed in an ad hoc manner over the past century. The new strategies for health, incorporating the targeting of activities, provide a new impetus to health promotion. The community development approach provides an opportunity to pursue a more people-centred, health-oriented strategy.

References

Battle, J. (1988) *Culture Free Self Esteem Inventory.* NFER – Nelson Publishing Co., Windsor.

Benzeval, M., Judge, K. & Whitehead, M. (eds) (1995) *Tackling Inequalities in Health. An Agenda for Action.* King's Fund Centre, London.

Billingham, K. (1989) 45 Cope Street: working in partnership with parents. *Health Visitor,* **62**, 156–7.

Bryar, R. and Fisk, L. (1994) Setting up a community health house. *Health Visitor,* **67**(6), 203–5.

Calnan, K. (1986) Maintaining health preventing illness: a comparison of the perceptions of women from different social classes. *Health Promotion,* **1**(2), 167–77.

Coulter, A. (1987) Lifestyles and social class: implications for primary care. *Journal of the Royal College of General Practitioners,* **37**, 533–6.

Davies, J. (1995) A study of family networks and relationships in community midwifery. In: *Practitioner Research in Health Care: The Inside Story* (eds J. Reed & S. Procter), Chapter 8, pp. 130–146. Chapman and Hall, London.

Farrant, W. & Russell, J. (1986) *The Politics of Health Information.* Institute of Education, London University. Cited in: Liddiard, P. (1988) *Milton Keynes Felt Needs Project. A Preliminary Study of the Felt Health Needs of People Living in Relative Poverty on a Milton Keynes Housing Estate.* Department of Health and Social Welfare, the Open University, Milton Keynes.

Fisk, L. (1992) *Bettws Community Health House: investigation into a new approach for health visiting.* TCV Project Report. TCV, Welsh Office, Cardiff.

Goodwin, S. (1988) *Whither Health Visiting?* Keynote Speech. Health Visitors Association Conference. HVA, London.

Graham, H. (1984) *Women, Health and the Family.* Harvester Wheatsheaf, Brighton.

Liddiard, P. (1988) *Milton Keynes Felt Needs Project. A Preliminary Study of the Felt Health Needs of People Living in Relative Poverty on a Milton Keynes Housing Estate.* Department of Health and Social Welfare, the Open University, Milton Keynes.

Parry, G. (1988) Mobilising social support. In: *New Developments in Clinical Psychology* (ed. N.W. Fraser), **2**, 83–104. British Psychological Society, John Wiley, Chichester.

Pound, A., Mills, M. & Cox, T. (1985) A pilot evaluation of Newpin: a home visiting and befriending scheme in South London. Summarised in the *October Newsletter of the Association of Child Psychology and Psychiatry*, 13–15.

World Health Organization (1978) *The Alma Ata Declaration.* Health for All, Series No. 1. WHO, Geneva.

World Health Organization (1991) *Community involvement in health development: Challenging health services.* Technical Report Series 809. WHO, Geneva.

Chapter 18

Understanding Depression in the Community

Harold Proctor, Patricia Davies and Paul Lewis

The history of community psychiatric nursing in Britain goes back to 1954 when nurses based in psychiatric hospitals started to follow up clients and families at home. Since then, the development of the CPN service has grown quickly to a point where CPNs are now commonly part of PHCTs (Simmons & Brooker, 1986). As such CPNs are now involved in the full range of mental health care from the preventive, through support of those with minor disturbances in their mental health, to support and intervention with those people with acute and chronic mental health disturbances.

Robertson & Scott (1985) found that the most common reasons for referrals to CPNs who were based in health centres were those of mood or affect, followed by behavioural and social problems. Government policy since the late 1980s has focused on the needs of people in the community who have long-term mental health problems (Welsh Office, 1989). This focus can cause conflict for CPNs in PHCTs where team members are more concerned with seeking help from CPNs for people with less severe conditions but who take up a considerable amount of their time (Repper & Perkins, 1995).

The impetus for this study was a noticeable increase in referrals from local GPs to CPNs. In particular, there was an increase in referrals of people who were described as 'depressed'. We noticed that some patients who were diagnosed as depressed by the GPs seemed 'unhappy' rather than depressed in the clinical sense. With these issues in mind, as a CPN team we decided to mount a study which addressed the following questions:

- How do CPNs decide that a patient is depressed?
- How do GPs decide that a patient is depressed?
- What would persuade a GP to refer a depressed patient to a CPN?
- What are the factors which precipitate the onset of depression in patients seen by CPNs?

This project was carried out by members of the Ystradgynlais Mental Health Team supported by the research nurse for Powys. Eight CPNs were involved in the project. Five were appointed as a team of short-term clinical fellows with TCV, for one day per week for six months.

Ystradgynlais is a small 'post-industrial' town situated on the southern edge of Powys, in the west of the TCV area. It is surrounded by a semi-rural area which includes many small communities served by several group practices. Three practices were included in the project. Five CPNs were based at health centres and three in the local Mental Health Resource Centre. We consider ourselves to be part of the PHCTs in the area. We have an open referral policy, accepting appropriate referrals from any source, but the majority of our referrals come direct from GPs. We each carry a generic caseload working with people with all types of mental health problems.

Defining depression and sadness

The classic medical text, *Diagnostic and Statistical Manual of Mental Disorders* (American Psychiatric Association, 1987:213), the DSM-III-R, describes mood disorders as characterised by: 'a disturbance of mood, accompanied by a full or partial Manic or Depressive Syndrome, that is not due to any other physical or mental disorder'. According to the DSM-III-R, therefore, depression is a mood disorder which can be associated with manic episodes. With this type of disorder, symptoms such as delusions and hallucinations are present. No other types of depression are described.

The International Classification of Diseases produced by the WHO (1978), however, recognises neurotic depression, and states that this has usually been precipitated by a distressing experience. Clare and Blacker (1987) believe neurotic depression is a term applied to milder depression. It may be stress-related, less severe and usually does not respond to antidepressant treatment. Snaith (1987) has argued that these milder types of depression are difficult to define.

Much research has investigated the relationship between life events and depression. Paykel *et al.* (1969) provide empirical evidence and identify eight events that have a significant link with depression:

- increased arguments with spouse;
- marital separation;
- change to new type of work;
- death of an immediate family member;

- serious illness of a family member;
- departure of family member from home;
- serious personal illness;
- substantial change in work conditions.

Further research carried out by Brown and Harris (1978) found that 'severe events' connected with loss and disappointment contributed to the cause of depression. Some events, such as bereavement, are more easily identified as precipitating depression. Parkes (1972) showed that, 14 months after bereavement, depression was evident in a sig nificant number of people who had lost their spouses. Unemployment is another area that has been well researched. Studies such as that of Liem and Liem (1978) found that unemployed men had a marked reduction in self esteem and a high incidence of estrangement from family and friends.

The percentage of patients who consult GPs about depression ranges between 12% and 42% (Zung & Magill, 1983). However, these figures are called into question by research which has shown that many GPs fail to recognise depression and often subject patients to lengthy, harmful and often costly investigations in order to explain the physical symptoms that these patients report (Zung & King, 1983). Where the depression is recognised, GPs often undertake care themselves, without specialist help, particularly in cases where the depression is mild. The rate of referral to psychiatrists has been estimated to be about 3 per 1000 (Paykel & Priest, 1992).

The study

To answer our research questions, it was necessary to obtain information from CPNs, GPs and clients. We organised our research in two parts.

Firstly we developed a semi-structured interview schedule to collect information from CPNs and GPs. We had some concerns about the length of time that the interviews might take, and about the amount of time that might be involved in transcribing and analysis. However, because we wanted to understand in detail the process of assessing and treating depression, we decided that obtaining qualitative data in this way outweighed the disadvantages (Crabtree & Miller, 1992). The interview schedules were piloted by interviewing one GP and one CPN from outside the study area. As a result of the pilot interviews, certain changes were made, so that the interview focused more clearly on the research questions posed. All interviews were audio-taped and each lasted for about thirty minutes. All seven CPNs and thirteen GPs who worked in the locality were interviewed.

The second part of the study consisted of questionnaires compl￰
by people who were new referrals to the CPNs during the cou￰
study. Fourteen clients completed a questionnaire.

Selected findings from the GP interviews

Certain themes emerged from the data enabling us to describe the pattern of the patient's journey to the GP and eventual referral to the CPN. When a patient visits a GP, the first important issue is the diagnosis. Often biological symptoms do not exist with psychiatric symptoms. The problem of making the diagnosis was explained by one GP as follows:

> 'If a patient who comes in and says "I have a chest pain when I walk up a hill, which is relieved by rest", by definition that is angina. I tend to use the same type of thing with a sort of list of seven or eight factors which perhaps go towards making the diagnosis of depression.'

This suggests that the process of identifying depression is much less precise than is the case in the diagnosis of physical illnesses such as angina. Sometimes depression is 'disguised' and not represented by a low mood, as this GP described:

> 'Someone may say "I have backache doctor" and you know you have done all the tests, they've had the works and they are still no better. Then perhaps this guy is depressed. I'm going back to a particular case ... about five years ago, a young girl, happily married or supposedly happily married, kept coming with backache, but nothing significant was found. The physio saw her and felt there was something to it. A CPN saw her as well, and she felt there was something going on here, and it is only now really that she's coming out with it that she is depressed.'

It seemed that it is often intuition, rather than objective assessment, that leads a GP to believe that a patient is depressed. One commented: 'By the time I've finished talking to somebody I have a feeling about whether they are coping or not, or whether they are happy or not.'

Recognising depression in general practice, therefore, appears to be fraught with problems – as much of the literature suggests (Zung & King 1983; Paykel & Priest, 1992). Although the GPs recognised that depression covers a great spectrum of symptoms, they tended to distinguish between two broad categories: sadness and depression (referred to by some GPs as 'exogenous' and 'endogenous' depression respectively).

One GP described sadness:

> 'They don't fall into classical categories, possibly of the early morning wakening, the loss of self esteem. A lot of these people are just cheesed off with problems at home, the kids are playing up. They are not having a lot of support from their spouse or from their own parents or the children's grandparents. Perhaps they have lost their job recently or are out of work. Lots of things like that, they are just unhappy.'

Depression on the other hand was described by one GP: 'Usually if they are not sleeping at night, they are constantly going to bed with a problem, loss of appetite, weight loss sometimes...'

Another describes it as: 'I think you usually have some of these other things, like lack of concentration, low self esteem, feelings of guilt or worthlessness, sleeping difficulties, either sleeping too much or early waking.'

For patients who are diagnosed as having depression, most GPs stated they would intervene by prescribing medication. One GP reported that. 'If I feel I can cope myself with the patient being depressed, I usually start them on medication and review them monthly and then decrease the dose accordingly.'

Most GPs indicated that in most instances of depression, medication would be prescribed and that CPN intervention would not be necessary. One GP, however, did mention that he would refer to the CPN, because he believed it was: 'good for them (the patients) to talk to someone at length, and you find that by talking they are actually improving. Then you don't need to give medication.'

The literature suggests that treatments such as cognitive therapy and behavioural therapy are helpful for depressed patients seen in primary health care. These approaches can be used separately or as an addition to medication (Paykel *et al.*, 1969). So, as the GP above suggested, CPN intervention can be extremely important in the early stages of depression.

Sadness, on the other hand, was treated differently by the GPs. In these cases, most GPs refer to the CPN quickly: 'If it is an exogenous depression and I feel there are external pressures that have to be delved into in some depth, I feel it is better done by the CPNs. They tend to have more time to spend.'

Time is the key point. GPs perceive patients who are sad as needing time to talk. GPs have very little time and so they refer these patients to CPNs:

'I would spend a little bit of time just talking to them. Even if I'm really busy I do try to let them talk a bit. And then I explain I don't have the time to discuss this, but if you would like to, there are a wonderful team of CPNs up the road, and then refer them on like that.'

These findings, taken from the interviews with the GPs, show that the patient's journey from the GP to the CPN is dependent on several factors. Depression can be missed by the GP and often misdiagnosed. A diagnosis of depression is often dependent on subjectivity rather than objectivity. The speed with which the person is referred to the CPN, therefore, is dependent on whether the patient is seen as bei 'depressed' or 'sad'. Time here is a factor; a person who is s requires time to talk will be speedily referred to the CPN.

who is 'depressed' will be prescribed anti-depressants in the first instance, only to be referred to the CPN at a later date if there is no improvement.

The patients' study

When the Community Mental Health Team were considering examining the reasons for the increase in referrals for 'depression', one possibility considered was that the increase was due to people who had experienced an increase in life events. Paykel *et al.* (1969) were probably the first to establish the relationship between depression and life events. Since then, many studies have supported the importance of life events precipitating the onset of depression (Brown & Harris, 1978; Costello, 1982; Campbell *et al.*, 1983). Brown and Harris (1978), studying women living in a working class area, further substantiated the role of life events, and added the concept of 'ongoing difficulties' as 'provoking agents' in depression. They identified ongoing difficulties as adversities which lasted two years or more.

Given the restrictions on our time, we decided that a questionnaire was the most appropriate method to obtain the information required from the sample of patients. The questionnaire design was based heavily upon the work of Paykel *et al.* (1969). Some changes and additions were made by the team to make the terminology more easily understandable, and some life events which were believed to be applicable to the locality were added; for example, redundancy.

It was important to establish the length of time prior to the onset of depression that the life event occurred and to whom: themselves, their partner, or a close family member. We also wanted to find out how stressful the individual had found the life event or ongoing difficulty.

During a three month period, new referrals from GPs were included in the study if depression was indicated in the referral letter. The questionnaire was administered at the initial assessment. A total of fourteen people met the criteria: ten female and four male. This was a lower number than expected. Clear conclusions could not be drawn, but some enlightening information was provided by the completed questionnaires.

A vast variation was found in the length of time from the onset of depression to the referral to the CPN service, ranging from two months to seventeen months. However, it was not possible to establish if lengthy delays were due to the patient putting off seeking help from the GP, or to the length of time between the initial contact with the GP and referral to the CPN. The number of life events (LEs) reported varied considerably. Most people identified between one and six LEs; one person reported as many as sixteen, while only one did not indicate any. Fewer ongoing difficulties were reported: six people said they had none, the highest number was four.

The 14 patients identified a total of 64 life events. These were placed into six categories (Table 18.1). A third fell into the 'Relationships' category.

Table 18.1 Percentage of reported life events for each category

	%
Relationships	33
Illness or death	20
Pregnancy or birth	17
Occupation	13
Legal involvement	9
Social circumstances	8
Total (= 100%)	64

Looking more closely at the relationships category, over half the events (11 out of 21) were found to be significant arguments with either a partner or close family member. We thought the serious illness/death category showed a high proportion of reported LEs, whereas the number of LEs in the 'occupation' category (including redundancy) were fewer than we had expected.

Previous research has indicated that individuals experience differing levels of stress for the same or very similar life events. Paykel *et al.* (1969) describe this as subjective impact. Table 18.2 shows there were some interesting differences in the level of stress reported for each category.

Table 18.2 Numbers reporting different levels of stress

Life event	Stress None	Slight	Moderate	Very high	Total
Relationships	5	1	4	11	21
Illness or death	0	1	2	10	13
Pregnancy	7	2	1	1	11
Occupation	1	2	1	4	8
Legal involvement	0	0	1	5	6
Social circumstances	0	2	2	1	5
Total	13	8	11	32	64

This shows that certain kinds of LE tend to be considered more stressful: arguments, illness, deaths and court appearances. In contrast other LEs such as pregnancy were on the whole found to be stressful or only slightly stressful.

As with life events, when reports of ongoing difficulties were analysed, relationships were the most often reported category. The level of stress was just as high for all ongoing difficulties, with 59% stating these to be very stressful.

Implications for PHC practice

The study showed that the GPs differentiated between sadness and depression, and that this differential diagnosis led to different referral behaviours. CPNs may have as much to offer the depressed as the sad. It is suggested that one way of exploring the different perceptions of GPs and CPNs would be through joint education sessions which could explore:

- the understanding of GPs and CPNs of what constitutes depression and sadness, possibly through the use of vignettes;
- devising and agreeing common diagnostic criteria;
- using depression rating scales in assessment;
- how to market CPN skills, so that GPs have a clear understanding of how CPNs can help with mental health problems;
- alternative interventions for depression which relate to life events or ongoing difficulties, for example, counselling or cognitive behaviour therapy;
- reducing the delay when GPs refer patients to the CPN team.

There is a need for further study of the association between depression and life events and ongoing difficulties, to establish whether or not the indications of this study are repeated elsewhere. If, for example, the high number of 'relationship' life events in referred patients is confirmed, then this will have clear implications for the skills required by CPNs.

The effect of the research on the CPNs

Several CPNs were involved in this study: not just those who were clinical fellows but also those who helped by completing diaries and by assisting clients complete the life events and ongoing difficulties questionnaire. For some of the participants, the depth of the research was new and so there was a consequent learning of the process. During the study individuals exercised skills they already had or developed new skills in: identifying appropriate methods, interview techniques, questionnaire construction, undertaking literature searches and critical appraisal of literature.

Some became aware for the first time of the vast amount of work that had already been undertaken on the subject of depression. Participants said that reading around the area had stimulated their interest in different aspects, raising issues which they hoped to follow up at a later date. Most participants found that the project stimulated their thoughts about depression. It generated questions such as: How did depression affect people? What were the causes? How was it best treated?

As the research went on, the results began to challenge assumptions which we had held prior to undertaking the project. For example, some had assumed that the high unemployment rate in the area was a contributory factor to depression, but this was not found to be the case in this sample. Participants also described an increasing awareness and concern of how gender can play a part in the identification of depression. Some said that they now ask clients more about life events, and had begun to think more critically about what actually constitutes a life event. They became aware that the same life event could affect different people in very different ways. One CPN said he understood more about life events that were normally perceived to be positive events. For example, getting married or planned pregnancy were very stressful for some clients and were significant in causing depression. Not all the effects of the research were positive. One CPN felt that the client questionnaires became an obstacle to her normal approach.

Undertaking the research as a group proved to be an interesting experience. It soon became clear that a co-ordinator was needed to help set deadlines and remind people about getting work in. Getting work in on time proved to be one of the major difficulties with the research. All the CPNs had busy caseloads and, although the time given by TCV in the short-term clinical fellowship was most welcome, it was not enough. CPNs inevitably missed deadlines and felt under pressure. Even without the project, they tend to work over their normal working hours on their caseload, so the research was an added pressure on their own time. However, all the participants enjoyed the experience and felt it had been of great value. Working as a group helped to further build team relationships, and respect for individuals grew as hidden talents and knowledge emerged.

The interviews with the GPs were also seen as a positive experience. They created an opportunity to sit down and discuss views about one subject for at least half an hour free from interruption – something that is unusual in busy PHCTs. This led to a greater understanding by the CPNs of the attitudes of the GPs, and a greater knowledge and understanding of the pressures of their job.

Overall it was felt that the project provided us with a unique opportunity to stand back and examine a part of our work in detail. We could see several ways in which we could change our practice and provide a better approach to the problem of depression.

References

American Psychiatric Association (1987) *Diagnostic and Statistical Manual of Mental Disorders (DSM-III-R)*, 3rd edn revised. American Psychiatric Association, Washington DC.

Brown, G.W. & Harris, T.O. (1978) *Social Origins of Depression: A Study of Psychiatric Disorder in Women.* Tavistock, London.

Campbell, E., Cope, S. & Teasdale, J. (1983) Social factors and affective disorder: an investigation of Brown and Harris's Model. *British Journal of Psychiatry,* **143**, 548–53.

Clare, A. & Blacker, C. (1987) *Depressive Disorders in Primary Care.* Tavistock, London.

Costello, C.G. (1982) Social factors associated with depression: a retrospective community study. *Psychological Medicine,* 12, 329–39.

Crabtree, B.F. & Miller, W.L. (eds) (1992) *Doing Qualitative Research. Research Methods for Primary Care,* **3**. Sage Publications, Newbury Park.

Liem, R. & Liem, J. (1978) Social class and mental illness reconsidered. *Journal of Health and Social Behaviour,* **19**, 139–56.

Parkes, C.M. (1972) *Bereavement: Studies of Grief in Adult Life.* Pelican, London.

Paykel, E.S., Myers, J.K., Dinelt, M.N., Klerman, G.L., Lindenthal, J.L. & Pepper, M.P. (1969) Life Events and Depression. *Archives of General Psychiatry,* **21**(6), 753–60.

Paykel, E. & Priest, S. (1992) Recognition and management of depression in general practice. *British Medical Journal,* **305**, 1198–202.

Repper, J. & Perkins, R. (1995) Targeting services for seriously mentally ill people: implications for community psychiatric nurses. In: *Community Psychiatric Nursing. A Research Perspective* (eds C. Brooker & E. White), 3(8), 127–53. Chapman & Hall, London.

Robertson, H. & Scott, D.J. (1985) Community psychiatric nursing: a survey of patients and problems. *Journal of the Royal College of General Practitioners,* **35**, 130–32.

Simmons, S. & Brooker, C. (1986) *Community Psychiatric Nursing: A Social Perspective.* Heinemann, London.

Snaith, R. (1987) The concepts of mild depression. *British Journal of Psychiatry,* **150**, 387–93.

Welsh Office (1989) *Mental Illness Services – A Strategy for Wales.* Welsh Office, Cardiff.

WHO (1978) *World Health Organization Manual of the International Statistical Classification of Disease, Forms and Causes of Death.* WHO, Geneva.

Zung, W. & Magill, H. (1983) Recognition and treatment of depression in a family medical practice. *Journal of Clinical Psychiatry,* **44**, 3–6.

Zung, W. & King, R. (1983) Identification and treatment of marked depression in general practice. *Journal of Clinical Psychiatry,* **44**, 365–8.

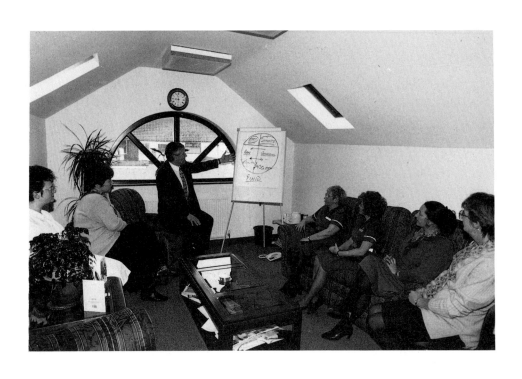

Section 5

Teamwork

In dividing these 22 chapters into five sections we have created some rather artificial distinctions: most of the chapters could have been included under any of the five headings. In particular, most of the preceding chapters have related in some way or another to teamwork. None, however, have focused specifically on teamwork. The chapters in this final section do just this.

The first chapter is concerned with the provision of maternity services by a team of four midwives and illustrates the ability of such a team to devise and undertake a quite considerable project designed to inform changes in the team's practice. The Amman Valley midwives first became aware of TCV through contact with some of the long-term clinical fellows on their initial visits to the practices to identify needs. Having discovered that TCV was a resource in the area, they asked TCV to help in the planning of a study day on continuity of care. Further discussions made them aware of the possibilities of becoming short-term clinical fellows. This, they realised, was an opportunity for them to undertake a study of the demand and need for continuity of care in the Amman Valley. It is widely agreed that mothers should be able to exercise more control through choice during pregnancy and childbirth and they were concerned to investigate the choices that mothers in the Amman Valley would make. Chapter 19 reports upon the findings of their survey.

Good teamwork is dependent upon good working relationships. What happens to these relationships, however, when teams are working under pressure? Chapters 2 and 5 have already touched upon this question. In Chapter 20 the results are reported of a systematic study of occupational stress in PHCTs in the TCV area. This used a standard and widely used indicator of occupational stress. It was found that stress levels were significantly higher than national standards. Approximately one in eight members of PHCTs in the TCV area had levels of stress characteristic of patients attending clinical psychology outpatient clinics. The study also shows that poor personal relationships are a major cause of stress.

One way of promoting good teamwork is through the provision of teamworking workshops. Chapter 21 reports upon an evaluation of a series of such workshops organised by Mid Glamorgan FHSA. This demonstrates the beneficial impact of participation. In addition it also investigates what practices might gain from follow-up support. The evidence is not conclusive but it does suggest that ongoing support is important in building upon the team reviews undertaken in the course of the workshops.

The last chapter comes close to encapsulating the TCV ideal. The PHCT based on a small isolated practice in West Glamorgan, close to a substantial opencast mining site, is undertaking a longitudinal study of childhood asthma. With support from TCV they were able to make contact with all four primary schools that serve their population, and then to undertake peak flow tests in the school playgrounds. When supplemented by questionnaires completed by parents, this data has enabled the team to establish a good asthma register upon which to run an asthma clinic, to challenge much of the stigma of asthma, and to develop other health educational initiatives with the schools.

The practice now has an important source of data upon which to monitor the health of the children and the potential effects of atmospheric pollution. But, from our perspective, the most exciting aspect of this project is that it represents a positive determination by a PHCT, in partnership with the community it serves, to raise the health of the practice population through concerted local action.

Teamwork, it may be argued, is not the natural behaviour of practitioners who have chosen to work outside institutions in community settings where they have more scope for independent practice. As this section shows, teamwork is not easy but, through a clearer understanding of the factors affecting the work of the team and the direction in which the team should be going, more effective teamwork can be achieved and through this more effective provision of care to the community.

Chapter 19

Providing Continuity of Care by Community Midwives

Rose Mary Marx

The Amman Valley lies in the west of the TCV area. It is a clearly defined rural area, mainly Welsh speaking, consisting of the main town of Ammanford and several small villages linked together by ribbon development. The total population according to the 1991 census is 15 744. The economy of the area has been seriously affected by the closure of coalmines in the 1980s.

In the 1940s, 50% of women having babies in the UK received full maternity care from GPs and district midwives. In 1948, however, the new National Health Service created a system of shared care between hospitals, local authority health services and the general practitioner executive councils.

In 1955 one in three babies were born at home. The Cranbrook Report (Ministry of Health, 1959) and later the Peel Report (Ministry of Health, 1970), however, recommended an increase in the hospital birth rate to 70% and 100% respectively, on the grounds of greater safety. Campbell and MacFarlane (1987) have since shown how this policy was determined with little reference to the evidence about comparative risk. The presumed greater safety of hospital care remains the tenet around which present day maternity services are organised, despite criticism from consumers that have been expressed since the 1970s. As a result of the trend towards hospital births, obstetricians became increasingly involved with normal childbirth. Both GPs and community midwives gradually lost their skills and confidence in providing maternity care in the intrapartum period (Tew, 1990).

This history is reflected at the local level in the Amman Valley. A purpose-built GP maternity unit with consultant cover was opened in

1951, obviating the need for home delivery. During the 1950s, up to 600 deliveries a year took place in this unit. The development of a consultant-led obstetric service in the 1970s, however, meant that fewer women were booked to have their babies locally and, resulting from a policy of centralisation of services in the 1980s, the Amman Valley maternity unit was closed. Following this the community midwifery service evolved with an emphasis on antenatal and postnatal care only, with on-call cover for obstetric emergencies or babies born at home unexpectedly. Women from the area presently give birth in consultant-led obstetric units in Swansea or Carmarthen, a distance of 16 to 25 miles or 30 to 60 minutes travelling time.

Four community midwives cover the Amman Valley area from an office in the Amman Valley community hospital. Three hold caseloads of approximately 80 births a year, an antenatal caseload that averages 45 women each at any one time. The fourth midwife is a relief midwife and all posts are grade G. Two of the midwifery caseloads are based on GP group practices within the town of Ammanford, and the third caseload is geographically defined, covering an area served by four separate GP practices.

The midwives work within a framework of shared care between the GP, midwife and consultant obstetrician. Midwife clinics are held at three GP practices where the midwife is seen as part of the PHCT. The satellite consultant antenatal clinics from Swansea and Carmarthen held at Amman Valley hospital are organised by the community midwives who are able to refer women directly to the consultant.

The pattern of antenatal check-ups is traditional. Women generally book early in their pregnancy, and tend to call in to see the midwives without appointment at their office if they have any worries or queries. Women are visited at least once at home in the last month of their pregnancy, or more often if there are problems or difficulty in travelling to clinics. In the postnatal period women are visited at home daily until the baby is ten days old, with a possibility of calling for up to a month if necessary. There is always good liaison with the health visitor before her first home visit at 11 to 14 days.

Impetus for change

Following the retirement of one of the midwives in 1991 and a subsequent change in staff, the team of midwives started to look critically at the service they were offering. It was felt that continuity in the antenatal and postnatal periods was good, but there was growing dissatisfaction about the lack of involvement with intrapartum care. The midwives felt they were not using their skills fully, and they were also aware that some women wanted their continuing support when in labour.

In Wales, the *Protocol for Investment in Health Gain: Maternal and Early*

Child Health (WHPF, 1991) preceded the publication of the English document *Changing Childbirth* (DoH, 1993) by two years. It was the Welsh document which we welcomed with enthusiasm since it gave us a rationale upon which to implement change. The Protocol requires improvements in the quality of the experience of childbirth to be measurable. It argues that more control for consumers through informed choice should be available, as should continuity of care with a known and trusted carer.

The Winterton Report (House of Commons Health Committee, 1992), on which *Changing Childbirth* was based, recommended the setting up of continuity of care schemes, and the re-evaluation of shared care. In the late 1970s the concept of 'team midwifery' had begun to emerge (Flint, 1979). Now, with the Winterton Report, midwives were beginning to be seen as the profession best placed and able to offer continuity of care and carer throughout pregnancy and childbirth.

These official guidelines published in the 1990s set out the principles, aims and objectives for the present organisation of maternity care. Within these documents a definite shift in ideology is evident, when compared with the official policy of the Cranbrook and Peel Reports and the Short Report (House of Commons Social Services Committee, 1980; Bryar, 1995). Women are now considered to be intelligent consumers who should be seen as partners with clinicians in the evaluation and audit of their maternity care.

In May 1992, we organised a study day in Llanelli on the theme of continuity of care. Midwives from the Rhondda and from Oxford were invited to talk about their continuity of care schemes, to an audience of 80 midwives mainly from South Wales. Following this successful day, we realised that if we were to establish a continuity of care scheme ourselves it would have to be individually designed for our area, and that local needs should be researched before any changes were made.

The project and TCV

Early in 1991 one of the team had met two of the clinical fellows from TCV when they were visiting one of the practices in the area and had learnt about funding for PHC projects that was available from TCV. We contacted TCV and formulated a research proposal. Following a number of meetings and discussion with our local managers we were seconded to the University of Wales College of Medicine for one day a week as short-term clinical fellows with TCV from June 1992 to August 1993. An experienced midwife was appointed on a temporary contract to enable us to undertake the research. Good team working was essential if this joint involvement was to succeed.

Despite the difficulties of combining practical casework with academic study, and the challenges of working together as joint clinical fellows, the individual and group benefits for the midwives of involvement with this study were many. Understanding the research process in depth was a learning experience in itself. This resulted in better knowledge about the application of research methods in general, and the scope and limitations of questionnaires, the method we used in the study, in detail. This has enhanced our understanding of social research and has directly promoted research appreciation.

The survey initiated active reflective practice amongst the team as we discussed the responses and comments from the women recorded on the questionnaires. This discussion led to a critical review of many aspects of professional practice. The self-reflection involved in this review led to the midwives having more appreciation of their own strengths and weaknesses and those of the other team members. Improved teamworking was achieved through undertaking the project both as a consequence of the reflection and the involvement in the project as joint fellows.

The survey

Our project was based on a descriptive survey which had three aims:

- to ascertain the need for a continuity of care scheme in the future, offering a 'domino' service (DOM-iciliary IN and Out, delivery in hospital by a known community midwife) and the option of a homebirth;
- to evaluate women's satisfaction with their maternity care;
- to audit current community midwifery practice.

Approval was obtained in October 1992 from the district ethics committee to enable selection of the sample from confidential midwifery records. The anonymity of respondents was assured.

Survey data was collected by use of self-completion questionnaires which consisted mainly of quantitative items with some open-ended qualitative components. The design of the questionnaires was based on the OPCS manual (Mason, 1989), questionnaires used in a study in the south of England (Melia *et al.*, 1991) and group discussion amongst the four midwives and with members of TCV.

The original questionnaire was piloted by a student midwife, who had extensive research experience prior to coming into midwifery. Ten women (eight who had given birth recently, two who were pregnant) were observed completing the questionnaires. Several parts of the questionnaire were either difficult to understand or misleading, and these were noted by the student. Individual questions were subsequently redesigned. Three questionnaires evolved following this pilot: two for postnatal respondents, one for hospital and domino births, the other for home births, and the third for all antenatal respondents.

A total of 167 women who had given birth between January and

September 1992 were included in the postnatal sample. Fourteen women were excluded: they had either moved from the area, had a neonatal death, stillbirth or cot death, or were young and in care. A total of 49 women (no exclusions) made up the antenatal sample. They were women resident in the area who were expecting a baby within three months of the survey, that is, between December 1992 and February 1993.

During November and December 1992, we distributed the questionnaires during antenatal and child health clinics, and by personal visits to women's homes. Completed questionnaires were posted, free of charge and without names, by the respondents to TCV in Cardiff, thereby providing reassurance to respondents about anonymity. At that time the women were either between 25 and 40 weeks pregnant (the antenatal sample), or had given birth to a baby between two and eleven months previously (the postnatal sample). By the end of February 1993, 45 women in the antenatal sample and 134 women in the postnatal sample had completed a questionnaire, a response rate of 82.9%. Within the postnatal sample there were 14 domino deliveries and 4 home births.

Coding of the responses was carried out by all the midwives, and the data analysed by SPSS (Statistical Package for the Social Sciences) with the help of an experienced researcher contracted by TCV. Interpretation of the results was undertaken by group discussion.

We faced one major problem in analysing the data. A definition of the domino system of care, which would help respondents understand what a domino delivery entailed, was not inserted in the right place in the questionnaire. Some women did not know that a domino delivery took place in a fully equipped maternity unit, and some women did not realise that it meant being cared for by a known midwife. Others equated a domino solely with a short postnatal stay in hospital.

Antenatal care

The findings of the study have been reported elsewhere (Marx *et al.*, 1993) and here some of the findings relating to antenatal experiences are discussed first, followed by some of the findings relating to postnatal and intrapartum care.

Table 19.1 shows that the majority of women from the postnatal sample were highly satisfied with the antenatal care they received from the community midwives. More women had had contact with midwives than with doctors, and they found the care being provided by midwives to be significantly more useful.

Women value the continuing relationship with their GP, but the high satisfaction with antenatal care given by the midwife supports the DoH's recommendation that a woman should be able to '... book with a midwife as her lead professional for her entire episode of care' (DoH, 1993:18).

Table 19.1   Contact and satisfaction with antenatal care received

	Contact with Midwife %	GP %	Hospital doctor %	Consultant or registrar %
No contact at antenatal clinic	5	11	21	27
Satisfaction				
Contact very useful	93	55	35	41
Would have liked more contact	26	14	15	26
Total (= 100%)	134	134	134	134

The antenatal care available in the Amman Valley area already fulfils the recommendation that '…the majority of maternity care should be community based and near the woman's home … obstetric and other specialist care should be readily available by referral from midwives or GPs' (House of Commons Health Committee, 1992, para 384). This situation is facilitated by the satellite consultant antenatal clinic being at the local community hospital, and being run by the community midwives. Overall 89% of the survey sample attended this clinic.

Postnatal care

The majority of women from the postnatal sample were very satisfied with the postnatal care from the community midwives. 97% of the women knew the midwife who made the first postnatal visit to her home, and 93% of the women were happy with the number of midwives who visited them at home. 96% felt the community midwives spent enough time with them postnatally, but 38% of the sample had felt that the staff in hospital were sometimes too busy to spend enough time with them. 21% of the women stated they were confused or worried by different advice in hospital after their babies were born, but only 5% were confused or worried at home.

It appeared that the midwives used their judgement well to assess how long a woman required support postnatally, since 79% of the sample felt that the number of days they were visited was 'just right'. 15% of primiparous women and 27% of multiparous women, however, felt that a daily visit was not necessary for ten days. The DoH (1993) recommends a flexible approach to postnatal home visiting, whereby the woman and her family determine the level of support that is required from the midwife. It was felt that the findings of the survey demonstrated that this form of individually tailored care was already being provided in the main, and that continuity of care is already central to the design of postnatal services in this area, as recommended by the House of Commons Health Committee (1992).

Intrapartum care

Disappointingly, 21% of the women thought the midwives were too busy to give them as much attention as they felt they needed during labour, and 10% thought they did not get enough attention during delivery. In retrospect we felt that the question which asked women how many midwives had looked after them in labour (a reason why women might prefer a domino delivery) was unclear, as responses did not give a true picture of the total number of carers a woman had been attended by throughout her labour. 85% of the postnatal respondents were happy with the number of staff who were with them during labour, and 86% were happy with the number of staff with them at delivery.

A wealth of data was obtained from the open-ended questions about satisfaction and dissatisfaction with the experience. Jacoby and Cartwright (1990) suggest that obtaining opinions about care is difficult, since general questions tend to elicit an expression of satisfaction, whereas more focused questions can determine preferences and obtain suggestions about the improvement of care.

The data obtained from women's comments is interesting in this respect: 77% of the sample felt that their preferences and wishes would be followed as far as possible during labour and delivery, 90% of the sample felt the midwives were attentive to their needs and available at all times during delivery, and 79% felt this was so during labour. Despite this apparent satisfaction, 64% of the sample chose to detail things they were particularly unhappy with. Analysis of this data for the purpose of this study was limited to grouping the responses together where a common issue had been identified or given importance.

Care and attention from midwives and from staff in general; wishes being met; being kept informed; and having adequate pain relief – these were the general areas about which 80% of the women made appreciative comments. Issues that women were particularly unhappy about were: lack of care and poor communication (by midwives), and certain aspects of the management of labour. A lesser number of comments were made about inadequate pain relief, not having wishes met and poor medical care.

Gaining responses in this way showed how the qualitative components of the questionnaire generated much data which could be used for further research, or indeed to formulate quantitative questions to obtain an indication of satisfaction about specific issues within maternity care; for example, adequate pain relief in labour and being kept informed.

When asked if they knew any of the midwives who looked after them during labour or delivery, only 22% of the postnatal sample said they did. 71% of the remainder said they would have liked to have known her. It seemed that some women felt 'let down' when their community midwife was not available to look after them in labour. In the section of the questionnaire asking what things they had felt particularly unhappy with, nine women made specific comment that they had not had the midwife whom they knew to deliver their babies.

Choosing hospital, domino or home birth

The themes for maternity care in the 1990s are continuity, choice and control (DoH, 1993). It is important in facilitating choice for women that they are aware of what alternatives are available. Most women were aware of the options of hospital or home delivery but it was necessary to discuss and define a domino service, in order for them to be aware that this was a third possibility. Simultaneously with the start of the survey a limited domino service was introduced in the Amman Valley. 60% of the women in the postnatal sample had discussed the possibility of a domino delivery, and 57% said they would have liked one.

There was evidence that the questionnaire not only served the purpose of the research but was, in itself, an awareness-raising exercise (see Chapter 15). In particular it was informing respondents that there were choices open to them, including that of a home birth – a service that up until 1991 was positively discouraged by community midwives in the Amman Valley. 52% of the respondents said that the possibility of a home birth had been discussed with them, and 16% said they would have preferred a home birth. Two-thirds of these women had discussed this possibility with their midwife, which suggests that discussion of the choice of home birth may increase the number of women who would be interested in it.

The final question of the postnatal questionnaire asked whether a hospital, domino or home birth would be preferred if the respondent were to have another baby. Correspondingly, the antenatal respondents were asked which they would prefer if the choice were available (Table 19.2).

The responses of the two groups are remarkably similar. When the two samples are combined 11% would prefer a home delivery and 43% a domino delivery. This indicates that 54% of the sample had a preference for community midwifery services.

Women having their first babies were less likely to choose home birth. Conversely, within the postnatal sample, the more children a woman had, the more likely she was to prefer a home birth. Over half of these women said that they were worried about getting to hospital when in labour. Primiparous women in the antenatal sample were

Table 19.2 Postnatal and antenatal preferences for place of birth

	Postnatal %	Antenatal %	All respondents %
Home	13	7	11
Domino	43	43	43
Hospital	38	45	39
Don't know	7	5	6
Total (= 100%)	128	44	172

more likely to want the domino system of care. The majority of women who would prefer a home birth were aged between 20 and 29 years. Women over 35 years of age were more likely to choose a domino, whereas it was much less likely that teenage women would.

It is interesting to note that, in regard to social class, the greatest demand for home birth was from women in the social classes I and II (professional/managerial) and social class V (unskilled manual). The greatest demand for domino delivery was from the social class III. Of seven trained nurses in the sample, all but one wanted either a domino or a home birth.

Those women in the postnatal sample who, after the birth of their babies, had been confused or worried by conflicting advice, or who thought that staff had been too busy to spend enough time with them, demonstrated an increased interest in home or domino delivery next time. This suggests that they believed that under a system providing continuity of care it would be less likely that staff would be too busy or that they would offer inconsistent advice.

In the postnatal sample, 14 women had a domino delivery and four a home birth. 13% of the sample, therefore, had continuity of care from a known midwife. Their comments about their experience were favourable. Women who had domino deliveries were asked about the advantages and disadvantages of this form of care. Thirteen of the 18 stated there were no disadvantages; two women were worried about the midwife becoming stressed by the demands made on her; two were uncomfortable travelling to hospital in late labour and one would have preferred to stay at home.

A total of 51 separate comments were made by these 14 women about the advantages of a domino delivery, some identifying the same factors (Table 19.3).

Discussion

Following the completion of this project we recommended that a continuity of care scheme should be implemented to meet the needs of

Table 19.3 Number of women mentioning the following as the main advantages of domino delivery

Good knowing the midwife	9
Staying at home for as long as possible	6
Continuity of care	4
Feeling relaxed and secure with the midwife	4
Midwife knowing individual needs and wishes	4
Knowing the midwife 'as a friend'	3

women using the maternity service in the Amman Valley area. The DoH has set the target that by 1998: '...75% of women should be cared for in labour by a midwife whom they have come to know during the pregnancy' (DoH, 1993:17). The importance of this target is certainly confirmed by this study. Women in the Amman Valley want to be cared for in labour by a midwife who is kind, understanding and attentive, who communicates well, meets their needs and respects their wishes. General satisfaction with the antenatal and postnatal services was demonstrated. The community midwives compared favourably with GPs and hospital care antenatally, and with hospital midwives postnatally.

However, in introducing continuity of care, adequate numbers of midwives are needed to maintain the quality of the antenatal and postnatal care that is provided at present. Such a scheme should be flexible enough to meet the needs of both the women and the midwives. Given the distance of the Amman Valley area from the maternity units in Carmarthen and Swansea, it would seem appropriate that a continuity of care scheme should be based in the local community, rather than in hospital as is being developed in some other areas. The necessity is demonstrated for clear and unbiased information about place of birth; with homebirth and the domino system of care being offered as realistic options.

Wraight *et al.* (1993) suggest that a team of midwives should be no greater than six. In order to make more time available for intrapartum care, it is important to review current patterns of antenatal and postnatal care, while at the same time ensuring that a service which women currently value is not jeopardized. A re-evaluation of the purpose and necessity of antenatal care must be undertaken in the context of shared care in the community. It is likely that there is antenatal 'over-surveillance' of women of low obstetric risk, and it may be that the purpose of much antenatal care is social support, better offered by a midwife than by a GP. A growing trend towards a short (6 to 12 hour) postnatal stay in hospital has implications for community services.

Women value continuity of midwifery care and they also value a continuing relationship with their GP throughout pregnancy and childbirth. Community midwives can no longer be satisfied with a situation where they are not involved in intrapartum care. Their experience must be in all spheres of midwifery. Given direct referral rights to an obstetrician, they are well placed to undertake the role of lead professional for the majority of women throughout their child-bearing experience.

The current trend in the education and professional development of midwives reflects the re-establishment of their autonomous practitioner status. This can best be facilitated from a firm foundation in the community, as acknowledged experts within PHC.

References

Bryar, R. (1995) *Theory for Midwifery Practice*. Macmillan, London.

Campbell, R. & Macfarlane, A. (1987) *Where to be Born? The Debate and the Evidence*. Oxford National Perinatal Epidemiology Unit, Oxford.

DoH (1993) *Changing Childbirth. Report of the Expert Maternity Group* (Chair, Baroness Cumberlege). Part 1. HMSO, London.

Flint, C. (1979) A team of midwives: a continuing labour of love. *Nursing Mirror*, **149**(20), 16–18.

House of Commons Social Services Committee (1980) *Perinatal and Neonatal Mortality* (Chair, Mrs R. Short). Second Report from the Social Services Committee, Vol. I. HMSO, London.

House of Commons Health Committee (1992) *Maternity Services*, Second Report (Chair, Mr N. Winterton). HMSO, London.

Jacoby, A. & Cartwright, A. (1990) Finding out about the views and experiences of maternity-service users. In: *The Politics of Maternity Care* (eds J. Garcia, Kilpatrick and M. Richards), Chapter 13, 238–55. Clarendon Press, Oxford.

Marx, R., Isaac, G., Jones, A. & Rowland, M. (1993) *Continuity of care from community midwives: a study into the satisfaction and future needs of women in the Amman Valley*. TCV Project Report. TCV, Welsh Office, Cardiff.

Mason, V. (1989) *Women's Experience of Maternity Care – A Survey Manual*. HMSO, London.

Melia, R.J., Morgan, M., Wolfe, C.D. & Swan, A.V. (1991) Consumers' views of the maternity services: implications for change and quality assurance. *Journal of Public Health Medicine*, **13**(2), 120–26.

Ministry of Health (1959) *Report of the Maternity Services Committee* (Chair, Lord Cranbrook). HMSO, London.

Ministry of Health (1970) *Domiciliary Midwifery and Maternity Bed Needs: Report of the Standing Maternity and Midwifery Advisory Committee* (Chair, Sir J. Peel). HMSO, London.

Tew, M. (1990) *Safer Childbirth? A Critical History of Maternity Care*. Chapman & Hall, London.

WHPF (1991) *Protocol for Investment in Health Gain: Maternal and Early Child Health*. WHPF, Welsh Office, Cardiff.

Wraight, A., Ball, A., Seccombe, I. & Stock, J. (1993) *Mapping Team Midwifery*. Institute of Manpower Studies, University of Brighton, Brighton.

Chapter 20

Measuring Occupational Stress in Primary Health Care Teams

Julie Slater

This chapter reports upon a study of stress in PHCTs (Slater, 1993). In particular it examines a paradox which the study revealed. The paradox is that, while results suggest that relationships with other people at work are one of the most significant sources of pressure at work, when questioned about other aspects of work, the same respondents cite work relationships as a source of job satisfaction.

Several contributions to this book have focused on the implications for PHC of the recent fundamental changes in the philosophical and cultural orientation of the NHS (see Chapters 2, 3, 5, 7, 11 and 15). These have placed immense pressures upon practices. It seemed possible that these constant shifts in policy and practice would reduce morale and job satisfaction. Initial visits to PHCTs in the TCV area confirmed that occupational stress, to some extent arising out of these changes, was a widespread concern.

The aim of this project was to provide descriptions and analyses of the stresses and strains of primary health care, and to determine the impact of these upon the well-being and job satisfaction of all role groups that might be members of the PHCT.

Methods used

Levels of occupational stress, job satisfaction and teamworking were measured in 43 general practices, comprising 310 PHC workers representing 11 role groups (Table 20.1). The Occupational Stress Indicator (OSI) developed by Cooper *et al.* (1988) was the principal

Table 20.1   Numbers of participants by role group

Receptionists	86
GPs	52
District nurses	41
Practice nurses	34
Practice managers	31
Health visitors	31
Administrative or clerical staff	15
Midwives	8
Community psychiatric nurses	7
Clinic nurses	3
Auxiliary nurses	2
Total	310

instrument used. It has been found to be valid with health care professionals (Rees & Cooper, 1990).

I was concerned both about the potential difficulties of gaining access to PHCTs and about the need to generate sufficient data to achieve the aims of the project; this meant that a convenience sample was appropriate. I invited all 155 practices within the TCV area to participate and the study is based on the 43 that volunteered.

Questionnaires were administered by myself to individual practices, usually during a lunchtime meeting. In many of the practices a key team member, usually a practice manager, took responsibility for ensuring a broad range of team members participated.

Administration of the OSI can be managed, without prior knowledge or qualification, by a team member (Cooper *et al.*, 1988). However, my experience suggests that, ideally, the administrator should be independent of the practice, and needs to liaise with a team member who has reasonable authority. PHC facilitators or health promotion officers would be well placed to act as OSI administrators. Above all, it is important that the use of the questionnaire is carefully planned and that the whole team is involved in consultation, from initial discussions through to follow-up. The use of the Indicator creates expectations amongst a team and changed perspectives and heightened expectations should be anticipated. Completion of the OSI can be seen as a first step in identifying problems within a team, and ideally should be followed up by an appropriate form of planned intervention at organisational or individual level. For this study, 34 teams provided sufficient data for the construction of individual team stress profiles. These allowed comparisons to be made with the normative data available from the publishers of the OSI. These teams received individualised feedback reports which included stress management strategies which were considered appropriate given their profiles.

Results

Table 20.2 shows that in comparison with the normative statistics for the OSI that are based on white collar and professional workers in industry (Cooper *et al.*, 1988), the PHC workers in the TCV area reported significantly greater pressure at work and higher ratings of mental and physical ill-health. They exhibited a greater tendency towards Type A (stress prone) behaviour, perceived themselves to have less internal control over their working environment, but used coping strategies to a greater extent. According to levels established by Rees and Cooper (1990), approximately 12% of the TCV subjects had stress symptoms of equal magnitude to patients attending clinical psychology outpatient clinics.

Table 20.2   Sources and effects of stress

	TCV group Mean	Sd	OSI norm Mean	Sd	Significant difference
Sources of pressure					
Factors intrinsic to the job	30	8	30	7	NS
The managerial role	35	10	34	8	5%
Relationships with other people	31	9	22	6	5%
Career and achievement	27	9	27	8	NS
Organisational structure and climate	37	11	35	9	5%
Home/work interface	30	11	25	9	5%
Mental ill-health	54	13	47	13	5%
Physical ill-health	30	10	22	7	5%
Total Type A characteristics	48	7	46	5	5%
Total locus of control	42	4	34	4	5%
Total (= 100%)	310		350		

Sd = standard deviation; NS = not significant

These findings indicate that people working in PHC are under substantially more stress than comparable groups. The health of a significant number is at risk. This has serious implications not just for their own well-being but also for the team as a whole. If absence through sickness is a common occurrence within a particular team, then this places still further pressure upon those at work. Thus there is a spiral of cause and effect which threatens the health of the community as a whole (see Chapter 5).

Sources of pressure

The Indicator is divided up into a number of sections. The sources of pressure section includes four scales that are predominantly concerned with team functioning: relationships with people, the managerial role, career and achievement, and organisational structure and climate. This section of the Indicator also measures pressure which is to do with the home-work interface and factors intrinsic to the job.

An examination of these various sources (Table 20.2) reveals that the greatest difference between the TCV group and the OSI norms is on stress due to relationships with other people: the mean for the TCV group is over one standard deviation higher than the norm. This source of pressure is characterised in the OSI by:

- lack of social support by people at work;
- conflict arising out of 'personality' clashes with others;
- lack of consultation and communication;
- dealing with ambiguous situations;
- lack of encouragement from superiors; and
- feeling undervalued.

Stress due to the home–work interface and to organisational structure and climate was also significantly higher in the TCV group and, to some extent, this also reflects pressure from relationships with other people (Table 20.2).

Job satisfaction

Responses to the job satisfaction section of the Indicator (Table 20.3) reveal that although the respondents in the TCV group showed more satisfaction than the norm group, this difference was not significant at the 5% level. The only significant difference within this section indicated that the TCV group were more satisfied with organisational

Table 20.3 Job satisfaction

	TCV group		OSI norm		Significant
	Mean	Sd	Mean	Sd	difference
Job satisfaction					
Achievement, value and growth	24	5	25	5	NS
The job itself	18	3	17	3	NS
Organisational design and structure	19	6	17	4	5%
Organisational processes	17	4	17	3	NS
Personal relationships	13	5	12	2	NS
Total (= 100%)	310		350		

design and structure. Although not significant, they were also more satisfied with work relationships than were the norm group.

This is the paradox referred to at the beginning of the chapter: given the stress that the TCV group were under from relationships with other people – lack of support, conflict, feeling under-valued, and so on – one might have expected significantly lower satisfaction in personal relationships.

A possible explanation lies in the differences between role groups (Table 20.4). There were four which were characterised by particularly high levels of pressure: practice nurses, district nurses, practice managers and midwives. With the exception of receptionists, these four groups all scored higher than the other groups on satisfaction. Thus, those groups that felt under the greatest pressure were also those that were most satisfied.

Table 20.4   Average scores for relationships with other people as a source of pressure and as a source of job satisfaction

| | As a source of | | Number |
	Pressure	Satisfaction	
High pressure and high satisfaction			
Practice managers	32.9	13.9	31
Midwives	32.7	14.3	8
Practice nurses	32.5	12.4	34
District nurses	32.4	12.9	41
Low pressure and high satisfaction			
Receptionists	28.4	13.2	85
Low pressure and low satisfaction			
CPNs	30.1	12.1	7
Administrative and clerical	30.0	11.5	15
GPs	29.8	12.3	52
Health visitors	29.5	11.8	31

Implications

In combining different strengths, skills and knowledge, teams play an important role in enabling people to accomplish more than individuals working alone and, if successful, team membership can be a source of satisfaction at work (Slater & West, 1995). In addition, team interaction facilitates learning and mutual support, thus contributing to personal and career development.

Nevertheless, however much satisfaction people may derive from teamwork, there are many obstacles and many things that can go wrong. There is enormous scope for stress when work relationships are considered, particularly when teams are multi-disciplinary. Although aspects of work such as overload or role ambiguity can cause anxiety, stress caused by interpersonal conflict is often the most intractable (West & Slater, 1995).

So does the experience of teamwork explain the paradox to which this chapter is addressed? Teamwork leads to both tremendous stress in personal relationships and, paradoxically, to potentially high levels of job satisfaction. Thus, how interpersonal relations are managed in teams is crucial.

Good conflict management can help overcome many of the barriers to good teamwork and can improve the organisational climate. Conflict within multi-disciplinary teams, such as exist in PHC, is inevitable and to a certain extent desirable. It can result from challenges to existing practices, and can provide the necessary stimulation or opportunity for new approaches to be introduced. Research has shown, however, that when teams react to conflict, they tend to attribute to individuals many problems which are due to team role or organizational factors (West, 1994). Interpersonal conflict in teams is often caused by organizational problems such as lack of structure or inadequate resources. Team members may focus on each other's behaviour and personalities to explain difficulties when the causes lie outside the team (Slater & West, 1995).

Consider two examples of conflict that were not uncommon in the TCV area. In PHCTs interpersonal conflict often involves GPs. Medical school training instils a powerful sense of individuality and GP training can serve to reinforce this. GPs receive little training in communication skills. This is poor preparation for working in teams. Also, the 1990 GP Contract has created extra work for doctors which in some instances has created role overload. Many GPs in the TCV area have delegated some of these extra organisational and managerial responsibilities to practice managers, and this has allowed the GPs to develop the clinical aspects of their own role. This has made their work more rewarding and satisfying. Taking practice management out of the hands of the GP has helped to reduce interpersonal conflict between these GPs and other team members. This seems sensible but, in these situations, the practice manager sometimes faces a difficult task in maintaining a smooth running team as opportunities for conflict are still numerous. For example, the history of relations between GPs and nurses is characterised by much conflict engendered by differences in power, status and authority. The reasons for this are deep seated and include differences in social class, educational background, gender and training. GPs often have limited understanding of the skills and knowledge of health visitors and district nurses. Conversely, nurses do not appreciate the ways in which GPs draw an income and invest in a practice, or the legal responsibilities they bear.

The second example of conflict within teams is that between community nurses, health visitors and practice nurses. The 1990 GP Contract has led to a marked increase in the number of nurses who are employed directly by GP practices (see Chapter 11). The rapidly developing role of the practice nurse has intruded into the territory of community nurses and health visitors, and some of the latter have become concerned about the erosion of their roles. Community nurses and health visitors have undertaken extra, specialised training and many have substantial experience of work in the community. Many feel threatened when newly appointed practice nurses begin to take responsibility for tasks which previously have been theirs. As organizational change continues to sweep through the health service, the roles of those employed by community trusts, such as community nursing and health visiting staff, may increasingly appear to be in jeopardy. This has served to further suspicion and hostility within PHCTs.

Thus, although the personalities of individual members are sometimes responsible for team conflict, many problems initially perceived to be personal are really functions of fundamental changes in structure and policy. When conflict arises in these situations, team leaders have to manage by helping members spend time exploring and clarifying each other's roles, recognising and accepting their differences.

Although mutual support within teams may not have a direct impact on team effectiveness, much research has illustrated the beneficial effects on the well-being of team members and therefore, indirectly, upon team effectiveness (Slater & West, 1995). Apart from efforts to sustain a good informal social climate within the team, other activities may involve more formal arrangements and longer term planning, such as arranging team away days, more formal training (see Chapter 21) or social outings. For example, one PHCT in the TCV area had an 'away day' every three months to which all team members were invited. Arrangements, such as a locum to cover for the GP, were made well in advance. After a pub lunch and a country walk, the team returned to conference facilities and enjoyed the opportunity to talk to one another away from the pressures of work. Another team marked every last Friday in the month with a surgery 'Happy Hour' from 6 pm onwards. Drinks and snacks were provided for those who wished to stay behind after work and all team members were invited. Such events give teams the chance to mix socially and to unwind after the pressures of the week.

Conclusion

This study has shown that PHCTs work under considerable pressure which threatens individual well-being. Poor personal relationships within teams have been shown to be a significant cause of stress. Paradoxically the results confirm that for most participants a major source of job satisfaction is their relationship with others. I suggest that the explanation for this lies in the co-existence within most teams of good team support – possibly within uni-disciplinary groups – and effective mechanisms for managing and coping with conflict.

The nature of multidisciplinary PHC demands a high degree of contact with people, so the quality of these relationships is crucial. Although the primary function of these teams is to provide health care in a community setting, it is important to recognise that teams have needs which must be met if they are to function effectively. The message of the study is that there is real value in managing team social relationships more effectively and in providing help in coping with pressure.

References

Cooper, C.L., Sloan, S.J. & Williams, S. (1988) *The Occupational Stress Indicator and OSI Management Guide*. NFER-Nelson Publishing Co., Windsor.

Rees, D.W. & Cooper, C.L. (1990) Occupational stress in health service employees. *Health Service Management Research*, 3(3), 163–72.

Slater, J.A. (1993) *Occupational stress in general practice*. TCV Project Report. TCV, Welsh Office, Cardiff.

Slater, J.A. & West, M.A. (1995) Satisfaction or source of pressure – the paradox of teamwork. *Occupational Psychologist*, **24**, 30–34.

West, M.A. (1994) *Effective Teamwork*. British Psychological Society, Routledge, Leicester.

West, M.A. & Slater, J.A. (1995) Teamwork: myths, realities and research. *Occupational Psychologist*, **24**, 24–9.

Chapter 21

Evaluating the Use of Workshops in Promoting Teamwork

Mary Ellen Brown

The debate about teamwork, and how to achieve it, is not new (Gilmore *et al.*, 1974; DHSS, 1981; Review of Community Nursing in Wales, 1987). What is new is the changed context within which it is taking place. The recent shift in emphasis of government policy to making PHC the basis of a preventive health care service has given impetus to the notion that teamwork among health care practitioners is necessary for the effective delivery of that service. In *Working for Patients* (DoH, 1989:14) the government attaches 'considerable importance to the strengthening of the primary health care team'.

Drury (1988) argues that, for the preventive health targets of government to become a reality, teamworking among PHC professionals is an essential pre-requisite. Tavabie *et al.* (1992) stated that teamwork is essential for members of PHCTs, not only to meet the needs of patients but also to meet government set targets for PHC. Waine (1992) has gone so far as to argue that effective PHC cannot be achieved without teamwork.

However, despite the strength of the argument that collaboration among PHC practitioners is necessary and desirable, the literature on teamwork continues to highlight the very real difficulties in achieving such a goal. The major obstacles to teamwork were summarised by the Review of Community Nursing in Wales (1987): a lack of shared premises, professional divisions among relevant personnel, misunderstanding of roles and objectives, and attitudinal barriers to co-operation among the different disciplines. Kohn (1983) observed that education and training in each of the disciplines involved in the delivery of PHC has concentrated on the requirements and tasks of that particular discipline, with the inevitable consequence that there is a low awareness of the skills and contribution that others can make to the care of patients. Gregson *et al.* (1991) concluded that there continues to be a low level of collaboration among PHC practitioners, some of the blame for which can be attributed to the fact that GPs, health visitors, district nurses and other PHC personnel come together with a heritage of working in an individualistic manner. Another reason postulated as an obstacle to teamworking is their different lines of managerial accountability (Review of Community Nursing in Wales, 1987).

In acknowledgement of these and other barriers to collaboration among PHC practitioners, a number of initiatives have taken place throughout Britain with the aim of promoting teamwork. In Wales, following the findings of the Review of Community Nursing in Wales (1987) the Welsh Office made available, for a number of years, funds to support implementation of the recommendations of the Review. In response to the need to improve teamworking in Mid Glamorgan, the FHSA set up a programme of workshops in the autumn of 1992 which were funded by this scheme. TCV was asked by the Welsh Office to assess the effectiveness of the programme in which nine of the 106 PHCTs in the county attended teambuilding workshops.

The study

Aims and methods

The aim of the study was to evaluate the effectiveness of the following two approaches to the development of teamwork:

- the use of workshops among PHCTs;
- the use of workshops with follow-up intervention visits.

Pre- and post-workshop questionnaires to follow the workshop were developed to enable a comparative evaluation to take place. Outcomes of the workshop courses were assessed by comparing the responses of participants before and after the courses, and by comparing data before and after the follow-up intervention visit. Information was also collected on the intervention visits to practices by TCV staff.

The effectiveness of the workshop programme as a method of promoting teamwork was assessed by comparing nine practices whose staff attended workshops with a control group of nine practices who participated in the study but who did not attend workshops. To establish whether intervention visits might have a role to play in promoting teamwork, the study also compared practices that were followed-up by an intervention visit after the initial data collection, with those who were not. Eight practices were selected for a follow-up intervention visit by TCV staff. Of these, four attended workshop courses and four were randomly selected from the nine study practice teams who did not attend workshops.

When the initial questionnaire was administered prior to the workshop course and the intervention visit, I was present to assist where a fuller explanation of questions was required. The follow-up evaluation questionnaire was self-administered three months after the workshop course or, in the case of the control practices, three months after the initial data collection (Brown, 1993).

Study population

Eighteen practices were selected to take part in the study by Mid Glamorgan FHSA. Nine GP practice teams were selected to take part in the three day workshops; four of these attended a residential workshop and five attended a non-residential workshop. The remaining nine practices did not attend workshops and acted as a control group. The practices came from the range of different geographical locations within the county.

The FHSA established a project team drawn from the FHSA and community units who specified the types of people who should attend the workshops from each team (Mid Glamorgan FHSA, 1993). Participating teams were requested to include at least five members drawn from attached as well as practice staff. Teams were encouraged to include as many members as possible from the following: at least one representative GP, a receptionist, a practice manager, a practice nurse, a health visitor, district nurse, community psychiatric nurse (CPN) or midwife and a social worker and nurse for learning difficulties. The teams who attended the workshops were also asked to include a patient representative on their team.

A total of 123 PHCT members completed the initial questionnaire, of whom 65 attended workshops. Ninety eight of the 123 completed the follow-up evaluation questionnaire. Of these, 49 had attended workshops; the remaining 49 had not attended the workshops and were members of the control group practices.

Results

Change following attendance at workshops

In order to assess the outcome of the workshop in terms of changes which might be attributed to the course, a number of questions from the first questionnaire were repeated in the second questionnaire. The main areas assessed for change were:

- perception of membership of the PHCT;
- understanding of roles;

- changes in teamworking activities (for example, objective setting, attending meetings);
- changes in attitudes to teamworking.

From the responses, it would appear that the workshops had an impact on several aspects of teamworking. First, the data indicated a general trend towards an extended perception of the membership of the PHCT. Seven participants (of the 49 attending workshops who completed pre- and post-workshop questionnaires) did not consider themselves members of the PHCT before the workshop: a CPN, a practice manager, a receptionist, a practice nurse, a midwife, a nurse for learning difficulties and a social worker. Of these only the practice manager did not consider herself a team member after the workshop.

There was an expansion in the number of different types of practitioners cited by respondents as being members of the PHCT. In particular CPNs, nurses for learning difficulties, social workers and midwives were more likely to be included.

Seven of the eight respondents who claimed not to understand the roles of some members of the PHCT prior to the workshop changed their response following the course. Of 15 respondents who thought that their own roles were misunderstood before the course, ten thought that their roles were understood afterwards.

The workshops had a significant impact on those respondents who stated before the course that the PHCT did not set objectives. Of these, 14 out of 18 changed their response to a positive one.

The workshops seemed to have had a major impact on the perception of the value of meetings. Twice as many respondents after the workshops as before saw meetings as providing time for discussion, ensuring uniformity of advice, and allowing the social aspect of teamwork to develop. Formal meetings had commenced in one practice, and increased in frequency in another participating practice.

Respondents were asked to assess teamwork within their PHCTs on a five point scale ranging from very poor to very good, and to agree or disagree with a number of positive and negative statements about teamwork on the same scale. Compared with the control group, participants who had attended workshops rated teamwork more highly on the second questionnaire. Respondents who had attended workshops showed a greater move towards agreeing with the positive statements about teamwork and in particular with a statement that teamwork increases job satisfaction.

Developing teamwork through intervention visits

Evaluating the effectiveness of intervention visits as a method of promoting teamwork was a further aim of the study. Of eight practice teams who received an intervention visit by TCV staff, four had attended workshops. The follow-up intervention visits occurred three months after the workshop course and, in the case of the control group, three months after the initial data collection. The objective of these visits was to assist PHCTs in the identification of obstacles to teamwork within their practices and, in the case of the workshop attenders, to assess with teams their ongoing needs following the course.

TCV staff involved in this process compiled a diary report of discussions and activities undertaken with participating practices. The diary reports indicated that the control practices identified the following key areas of concern which merited further discussion or support:

- conflict arising from lack of understanding of roles, in particular the roles of health practitioners not based in the practice, such as the health visitor;
- the need for improved communication between members;
- difficulties in arranging meetings;
- improving the usefulness of meetings.

The instigation of PHCT meetings was an outcome of the intervention visit to one of the control practices, with the date of the first ever such meeting in the practice being set during the visit. Among the workshop attenders, issues arising out of the workshop, such as how to involve all team members in setting standards of care, and how to continue to develop a collaborative approach among PHCT members, were discussed.

Evaluation of the intervention took place by analysis of the responses to questions on the evaluation questionnaire regarding:

- whether participants found the intervention visit useful;
- whether participants felt that their PHCTs would benefit from, or had a need for assistance in, developing teamwork.

Of the 33 PHCT members whose practices had received the intervention visit two in three found it useful and 22 responded that there was a need for support in developing teamwork activities. A slightly higher proportion of the control group (14 out of 19), compared with the workshop attenders (8 out of 14), thought that their PHCT would benefit from support. This may reflect a perception by the workshop attenders that the course itself was sufficient in facilitating the development of teamwork. However, it could be argued that the fact that over half of the workshop attenders stated that there was a need for further assistance indicates an unmet need for support (see Chapter 2).

Because of the short timescale over which the intervention visits took place, and the small sample size, it is not possible to draw firm conclusions about the effectiveness of this approach to developing teamwork among PHC practitioners. However, the majority of the study population who had received visits identified a need for support in developing teamwork. In addition, the fact that the problems identified as meriting attention were in keeping with impediments to team-working widely acknowledged in PHCT literature (DHSS, 1981; Review of Community Nursing in Wales, 1987) would indicate that a protocol for working with individual practice teams to help them address their needs, might help in promoting teamwork.

Considerations of the study

The preceding discussion suggests that the workshops course had an impact on a number of areas of teamworking activity. However, there are a number of points which merit consideration when assessing the results of this study:

- The eighteen participating practices were selected by the FHSA and as such are not necessarily a representative sample of other practices within the county.
- The evaluation took place over a short timescale, and as such may not have allowed sufficient time for evidence of change to emerge.
- Change may have occurred independently of the workshop courses.

Nevertheless the actual process of participating in the workshop influenced outcomes. For example, the workshop programme called for participating teams to develop 'action plans' aimed at responding to health needs of the practice population and there was a noticeable increase in the number of participants reporting in their second (evaluation) questionnaire that their team set objectives following the workshop. At a 'Teamwork in Primary Care' conference held in Mid Glamorgan 18 months after the first workshop course, a number of practice teams who participated in the course reported ongoing beneficial effects from their attendance. This would indicate that a workshop programme may have long-term value for triggering the process of developing collaboration between PHC practitioners beyond the initial intervention.

The actual process of participating in workshops may also have value in itself, merely by offering busy practitioners protected time for discussion and reflection. This might also be true of a programme of intervention visits to practices aimed at helping teams identify their needs and adopting a problem-solving approach to meeting these needs. The facilitation of teambuilding within the practice setting through such intervention visits might be useful either in conjunction with, or instead of, a programme of workshops held in unfamiliar surroundings.

Conclusion

Central to this study has been an assumption that a collaborative approach among PHC practitioners is essential for the effective delivery of PHC. The new demands that are being made on PHC, in particular with the emphasis placed on achieving preventive targets, has given greater impetus to the need to utilise the skills of all the different members of the PHCT. The shift of focus to health promotion and the increasing emphasis on care of patients with chronic diseases offers opportunities for GPs to delegate some of their workload and develop protocols with nurses and other PHCT members. Such an approach, in which the skills and contributions of different PHCT members are recognised and valued so that the greater demands on PHC can be met, may of necessity result in improved teamwork. The shift to fundholding may also result in better collaboration among PHC practitioners, if this leads to the skills of different practitioners being valued and their status being increased.

However, collaboration among PHC professionals continues to be problematic. It is likely that even if there are changes in the organisation of PHC that should, in theory, lead to greater collaboration among practitioners, the need for training in teamwork, such as workshop courses, will almost certainly remain a necessary way of promoting such co-operation. It may be that the ethos of teamwork conflicts with the desire for autonomy which motivates many GPs and nurses to choose to work in PHC in the first place. Any activity which brings such practitioners together, with a view to breaking down such barriers, is worth investigating. As an approach to developing teamwork, the use of workshops appears to have some impact. Although it is difficult to draw firm conclusions about the effectiveness of the intervention visits it would appear that such an approach to promoting teamwork is a useful adjunct to a workshop programme.

References

Brown, M. (1993) *Final Evaluation of Primary Health Care Team Workshop Project.* TCV Project Report. TCV, Welsh Office, Cardiff.

DHSS (1981) *The primary health care team.* Report of a joint working group of the Standing Medical Advisory Committee and the Standing Nursing and Midwifery Advisory Committee. HMSO, London.

DoH (1989) *Working for Patients.* HMSO, London.

Drury, M. (1988) The White Paper and the practice team. *Practice Update,* **36**(10), 2428–31.

Gilmore, M., Bruce, N. & Hunt, M. (1974) *The Work of the Nursing Team in General Practice.* Council for the Education and Training of Health Visitors, London.

Gregson, B., Cartilidge, A. & Bond, J. (1991) *Interprofessional collaboration in primary care organisations.* Occasional Paper 52. Royal College of General Practitioners, London.

Kohn, R. (1983) *The Health Centre Concept in Primary Health Care.* WHO, Copenhagen.

Mid Glamorgan FHSA (1993) *Primary Health Care Team Workshop Project Report.* Mid Glamorgan FHSA, Pontypridd.

Review of Community Nursing in Wales (1987) *Nursing in the Community: A Team Approach for Wales* (Chair, Mrs N. Edwards). Welsh Office, Cardiff.

Tavabie, A., Sparks, R. & Dickson, J. (1992) Primary health care team workshops – a new approach to planning and team building. *Postgraduate Education for General Practice*, **3**(3), 213–17.

Waine, C. (1992) The primary care team. *British Journal of General Practitioners*, **42**, 498–9.

Chapter 22

Researching the Prevalence of Childhood Asthma in a Practice Population

Duncan Williams and Beth Griffiths

This chapter describes the conception, planning, undertaking and early results of a research project being mounted in one small practice. The project was designed to accomplish certain aims and to answer specific questions regarding one aspect of work of a Valleys-based PHCT. As is evident, the chapter is written in two parts.

In 1991, I (Duncan Williams) took up a position as a single-handed GP in the upper Swansea Valley in West Glamorgan, in the west of the TCV area. The practice then consisted of 3600 patients with three part-time receptionists, rented accommodation in a converted café, and a number of dedicated attached staff: district nurse, health visitor and midwife.

Historically, the practice had responded to illness in the area without worrying about health needs or anticipatory care. As a result the prevailing attitude to health was one of 'the doctor knows best and the doctor has (or should have) the pill for every ill' – usually in the form of a prescribed antibiotic! There was very little information recorded in the GP records other than hospital letters. My predecessors had set up a limited age/sex register for the over-75 health checks, but most family planning, contraception and smear testing was done at the local DHA clinic.

As a new broom sweeping clean, my first few months in practice were not without their problems. A new appointment system was established and I refused to see patients without appointment unless they really were ill. This led to some disgruntled customers leaving the practice. Also, when I asked patients to attend surgery rather than have housecalls, a few letters were posted to the local MP. This led to some ill-conceived comments by the MP in the local paper. This gave me an ideal opportunity to reply in full to my critics with a breakdown of all the positive changes which had been introduced: the appointment of a full-time practice nurse and a practice manager, longer surgery times with the doctor available for longer hours, health promotion clinics and an effective PHCT. Following this public exchange, I detected a change in attitude in the practice population.

At about this time I began to think of ways of increasing the involvement of the practice in the local community, and of ways of breaking down the prevailing attitude of demand-led rather than needs-led health care. At the same time I received information from the local FHSA that TCV would be interested in funding projects involving teamwork in PHC.

The prevalence of asthma

Since starting in the practice, I had been struck by the high prevalence of undiagnosed childhood asthma and by the high level of parental anxiety and occasional anger relating to this. I had come across similar problems in previous practice in urban South Wales and in the southeast of England. However, the sheer number of cases in this part of the Valleys seemed exceptional. I started to question my own diagnoses and decided that one way to answer my uncertainties would be to establish a project with the objective of measuring the true prevalence of childhood asthma in the area. This project seemed to lend itself to several other aims too:

- It would promote preventive medicine in the practice.
- It would increase the profile of the (new) practice within the community.
- It would de-stigmatise an important and common childhood illness.
- It would educate parents about asthma.

In 1992 I appointed Beth Griffiths, a nurse and midwife, to the post of 'practice health facilitator' with responsibility for health planning, health promotion, audit and research within the practice. With her, I developed the methodology for the project.

Early on, we discounted the idea of measuring peak flow rates by calling children to the practice itself. Available space in the converted café was rapidly diminishing and so we decided to approach the four local primary schools. By enlisting their support we would help achieve another primary aim: that of bridge building within the community.

TCV was contacted and was immediately and enthusiastically supportive. We were advised by TCV on how to turn our ambitions into a fundable project and, following agreement, I was appointed a short-term clinical fellow. A draft outline of the aims, methods and anticipated results was prepared and put before the local ethics committee, which gave its approval for the project to go ahead with the proviso that written agreement of school governing bodies be obtained.

The seven objectives of the project were as follows:

(1)   To measure the prevalence of asthma in the study area.
(2)   To identify cases of undiagnosed asthma.
(3)   To increase awareness and reduce fear and stigma in asthma.
(4)   To forge links between the PHCT and local schools.
(5)   To assess the value of measuring peak flow rate against body mass index as a diagnostic tool.
(6)   To look at possible local contributory factors in asthma.
(7)   To set up cohorts for long term study.

First, in consultation with local paediatric consultant colleagues and with the schools, a questionnaire, along with an explanatory letter and consent form, was designed and distributed to the parents of approximately 300 local primary schoolchildren. The most difficult aspect of this was the translation of the questionnaire into Welsh. I deliberately chose not to use an existing standard asthma questionnaire as I felt this would detract from the originality of our project.

Second, the actual exercising and measuring of peak flow rates, heights and weights of the children was carried out in each of four local primary schools on one day. Pupils whose parents had consented were first weighed and measured for height. Then their resting peak flow rate was measured. Next they were exercised. This consisted of six minutes of free running and then serial peak flow rate measurements taken at 5, 10 and 15 minutes. At one school, photographs were taken and a local Welsh language TV company turned up to film the exercise – real community involvement! A video tape copy of the film is now in the practice library.

Third, the results were analysed both quantitatively and qualitatively. What this revealed was that approximately 33% of children had some evidence of asthma on the basis of the questionnaire and/or the exercise testing.

Teamwork in the community

When I (Beth Griffiths) joined the practice, the wheels were already in motion for the project. I was responsible for the fieldwork and the organisation that went with it. I consulted all members of the PHCT for help with different aspects. For example, one of the receptionists had close links with one of the schools and so she gave me guidance in approaching it. The practice manager had links with the local television company and she suggested that we should give the project media coverage. These numerous discussions helped the staff feel that the project belonged to them as a practice. We all shared the same objective

– an exciting research project that would put the practice on the map. All the staff working in the practice live in the locality and so we felt we would benefit personally from the medical and social aims of the project. We all became very proud of it.

The shared objective for the team was very important, but so too were the links that the project forged with the local primary schools and with the community itself. Making links with the local schools was an interesting experience. I found that those teachers who appeared less enthusiastic at first were the most supportive in the end. Initially, dealing with members of a different professional discipline unrelated to health was strange as we seemed to have such different objectives. But we soon came to realise that working closely together has many benefits for ourselves and for the children. We have helped the teachers understand more about asthma and its medication, and they have helped us to communicate better with the children. Developing from the project I have now devised a health education programme for the schools on various topics that promote healthy lifestyles. This has been approved by each Board of Governors. We, as health professionals, are no longer strangers to the classroom and the teachers welcome this. They often take the opportunity to ask about problems they have with children.

The children found the project very exciting, particularly as it involved being released from classwork to run around the yard for six minutes. It was to our advantage to go out to the schools and to meet the children on their familiar territory. It has helped them to relate to us as 'people', not as a nurse or doctor, and we are not now associated solely with illness and pain. A good relationship with children is very important: not only are they the adults of the future, but they can be very influential at home. This influence has been important in the destigmatization of asthma and in the education of parents. The opportunity to chat to the children about asthma generated some interesting questions and discussions, and the children with diagnosed asthma were hailed hero of the moment.

The powerful influence that children have on their parents is used by commercial advertisers and it can be seen in almost every aisle in every supermarket. We as health promoters must also use their influence to promote health, to get children to be health promoters themselves. One of the competitions we organised for the schools was to design a T-shirt to promote stopping smoking. The prizes were the successful printed T-shirt itself and so the children now wear this in the village, thus helping to reinforce our message about smoking.

Conclusion

The project was a resounding success. Asthma is no longer a feared diagnosis in this area. Our asthma clinic is well attended by informed parents and children alike. It is supervised by our practice nursing team who are now well known to the children, having been invited back to talk on other health issues such as diet, smoking and drugs. Findings have been presented to the local faculty of the Royal College of General Practitioners and to a local research presentation evening for the University of Wales Swansea. Both presentations were well received. We feel that the teamwork resulting from the project is one of the reasons it has been such a success. It has helped us get together as a PHCT.

Some of the objectives of the project (numbers 5, 6 and 7 listed above) have yet to be completed. TCV provided the resources to establish this as an ongoing project. What are now needed are further funds and time to sustain it. We hope at some future date to complete the analysis of the data generated in 1991 and 1992 by the asthma project, and perhaps to repeat the process and to evaluate other aspects of practice along similar lines. Certainly, our first experiences of practice-based research have been encouraging and, as we write this chapter and feel all enthusiastic again, we only wish we had the time!

Appendix 1

The Staff of Teamcare Valleys

Director
Dr Brian Wallace

Senior Lecturers
Miss Rosamund Bryar
Dr Bill Bytheway
Dr Peter Edwards
Dr Helen Houston

Lecturer
Mrs Stephanie Williams

Clinical Fellows (long-term)
Dr Michela Amann
Ms Mary Ellen Brown
Mrs Gwen Davies
Dr Peter English
Mrs Jennie Gill
Dr Sian Hunt
Mrs Rachel Pritchard
Ms Julie Slater
Miss Andrea Thomas
Dr Carl Venn
Dr Diane Wallis

Clinical Fellows (short-term)
Ms Kath Berney
Mrs Lisa Coles

Mr Alan Cooper
Ms Jane Czyrko
Mrs Karen Davies
Mrs Lyn Fisk
Mr Peter Ganesh
Dr Brian Gibbons
Ms Pamela Griffiths
Mrs Patricia Harwood
Dr Edna Hayes
Mrs Anna Hitch
Dr Chris Hoddell
Ms Gwyneth Isaac
Ms Ann Jones
Dr Robert Jones
Mr Paul Lewis
Ms Rose Mary Marx
Mr Paul Morgan
Mr Harold Proctor
Mrs Christine Rees
Ms Meinir Rowland
Mr Rolf Schulz
Dr Ajay Thapar
Dr Duncan Williams

Research Officers
  Ms Carolyn Eason
  Mr David Middleton
  Ms Sandra Parsons

Administrative Assistants
  Miss Jill Allen
  Mrs Julia Watkins

Secretaries
  Miss Jayne Broad
  Mrs Joanna Brown
  Mrs Sue Elsam
  Miss Christine Jefferson
  Mrs Judith Owttrim

Clerical Assistant
  Mrs Karen Bibey

Appendix 2

The Location of the South Wales Valleys in the UK

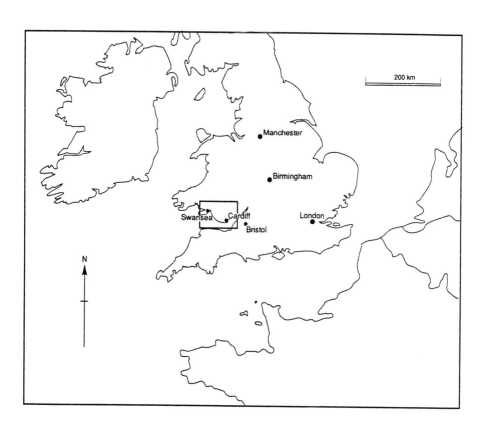

Appendix 3

The Teamcare Valleys Area

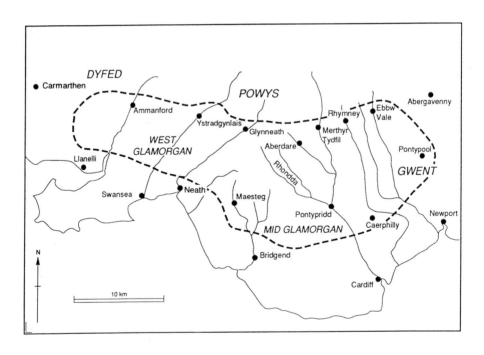

Index